The Strong Bones Diet

The
Strong Bones Diet

The High Calcium
Low Calorie Way
To Prevent Osteoporosis

By Lois Goulder
and Leo Lutwak, MD, PhD

TRIAD PUBLISHING COMPANY   GAINESVILLE, FLORIDA

Published and distributed by
Triad Publishing Company, Inc.
1110 Northwest Eighth Avenue
Gainesville, Florida 32601

Library of Congress Cataloging-in-Publishing Data
Goulder, Lois.

The strong bones diet.
1. Osteoporosis--Diet therapy. 2. Osteoporosis--
Prevention. 3. Osteoporosis--Diet therapy--Recipes.
4. High-calorie diet. 5. Low-calorie diet.
I. Lutwak, Leo. II. Title. (DNLM: 1. Calcium,
& control--popular works. WB 428 G697s)
RC931.073G68   1985   616.7'1   85-16459
ISBN 0-937404-20-9

Printed in the United States of America

The nutritional content of the recipes (Chapter 10) were calculated by the HVH-
CWRU Nutrient Data Bank at Case Western Reserve University in Cleveland, Ohio,
which includes more than 3,000 foods in its computer bank.

Calcium and calorie contents of foods throughout the book are taken from   U.S.
Dept. of Agriculture Handbook 8-11, "Composition of Foods: Vegetables and Vegetable
Products," revised 8/84, and "Value of Foods, Home and Garden Bulletin #72, revised 4/81.

**Major changes should not be made in the calcium intake of your daily
diet without first consulting your physician. This includes increases in
certain foods, as well as calcium supplements.**

TO THE PIONEERS whose research in the 1950s and 1960s on the use of calcium in the prevention and treatment of osteopososis is just now being recognized:

Goran Bauer, MD, PhD
Lennart Krook, DVM, PhD
William Neuman, PhD
B. E. C. Nordin, MD, PhD
G. Donald Whedon, MD

CONTENTS

List of Tables

RECIPE CONTENTS

BETTER BONE HEALTH
WITHOUT PILLS

BUSY AMERICAN WOMEN who skillfully juggle jobs, motherhood, and countless other responsibilities need to take good care of their bones so that osteoporosis will not prevent them from leading active vigorous lives when they are older.

Yet every single day millions of women take unnecessary risks with their bone health by not consuming enough calcium in the foods they eat. Zealous calorie-watchers who drastically limit food selections may not realize that weight loss is often accompanied by nutrient losses, whose effects may not be felt for many years.

One effect of obsessive dieting may be harmful calcium deficiencies and weakened bones. That's why women who watch their waistlines need to pay special attention to their food choices, making sure that the minimal-calorie foods contain the maximum amount of healthful vitamins and minerals, including enough calcium.

Why not just take a pill?

In response to the alarming TV commercials that depict wrinkled, hunch-backed old women suffering from osteoporosis, many women have started to take daily calcium supplement pills, purchasing them at the drugstore without a prescription. Later, if they develop abdominal discomfort, constipation, or even kidney stones, many regret that they did not consult their physician. *Calcium supplement pills should never be taken without consulting a physician.*

Some calcium supplements contain vitamin D, which is necessary in the process of calcium absorption. However, some of these supplements contain so much vitamin D that if you take enough pills to fulfill your daily calcium requirement, your vitamin D total will far exceed the U.S. RDA recommendation of 400 IU. Vitamin D in excess of 1,000 IU per day may, in itself, result in bone loss and other harmful effects.

Many physicians do, of course, recommend calcium supplements for their patients, expecially in those age groups with increased calcium needs. Others recommend that patients try to meet a major portion of daily calcium needs by eating a wide variety of calcium-rich foods.

The Strong Bones Diet was written for those who want to rely less on pills and more on foods. There are advantages to getting your calcium from foods instead of pills. Bone health depends not only on calcium, but on many other nutrients that are contained in different kinds of foods.

High calcium foods contain a wide variety of other minerals and vitamins necessary for good health.

High calcium vegetables are excellent sources of fiber, which makes you feel full, so you are satisfied to consume fewer calories. Fiber also may help prevent cancer of the colon.

Foods give you energy; pills don't.

You may forget to take one or more pills throughout the day, but your "growling" stomach always reminds you to eat.

If you don't have to worry about gaining weight and don't have any other dietary restrictions, you may already be eating the wide variety of foods that provide the nutrients necessary to keep your body healthy. But if you do limit your diet for any reason, your choices need to be informed ones. Once you are able to identify the foods that are the best sources of calcium, you will find it easy to include them in your daily diet. Then you can set your own calorie boundaries to suit your individual needs.

Unlike many diets that stringently restrict food choices, *The Strong Bones Diet* offers a wide variety of high calcium taste adventures. You'll discover that you can increase your intake of calcium without gaining weight, so long as you "trade off" high calorie foods that are low in calcium for high-calcium foods that are low in calories. For example, you could pass up a glazed doughnut (235 calories) at the office in the morning and later snack on an ounce of Swiss cheese (110 calories). The cheese provides 30 percent of the U.S. RDA for calcium, while the doughnut has less than 2 percent calcium.

The Strong Bones Diet provides authoritative medical information, up-to-date data on the calcium and calorie content of more than 1,200 brand-name foods, a special fast-foods restaurant calcium guide, 60 high calcium recipes including snacks for kids, and even a gardening section on growing high calcium vegetables in your own backyard. You will learn how to make healthful food choices — small changes now, that can later result in big changes in the health of your bones.

PART I

HOW TO PREVENT OSTEOPOROSIS

1

IMPROVING THE ODDS
AGAINST OSTEOPOROSIS

Laura's Story

"DO YOU HAVE your Golden Age card with you?" The pretty young clerk at the checkout counter smiled at Laura as she pointed to the sign above the cash register.

"You can get ten percent off the purchase you just made if you have your card," the clerk added, smiling brightly.

Laura didn't smile back. She was furious. Who was this young snip? How could she possibly have mistaken Laura for a sixty-five-year-old woman?

Laura believed — at least her friends kept telling her — that she still didn't look her age, which was fifty-five. Laura had always looked younger than her years, due in part to her vigorous dieting and her hairdresser's skill in keeping her reddish-blond hair the same color it had been when she was twenty.

Laura's hand trembled as she took a ten dollar bill out of her purse.

"You ought to get an eye examination. Can't you see I'm not old enough to have a Golden Age card?"

The clerk's face flushed. She muttered a meek "I'm sorry," and busied herself taking the change out of the cash register. Laura snatched up her package and stormed out of the store. She kept her head down as she walked, blinking away the tears that filled her eyes, knowing full well that the "dowager's hump" on her upper back and the recurrent pain in her spine kept her from standing tall and straight and in fact made her look old.

Until recently, Laura never suspected that years of bone loss had made her skeleton weak and fragile, and that she had, in fact, lost enough bone to have had fractures of her spine. Even when she had two

15

early signs of osteoporosis, she did not recognize them. Now she berates herself for not asking her doctor about the nagging backache she had for no apparent reason; instead she told herself she needed a new mattress. The other clue had come during her last medical checkup. While she was being weighed and measured, the nurse had commented, "You're about an inch and a half shorter than you were last year." Laura realizes now that she had heard only what she wanted to hear: "You've lost five pounds," and she had smiled with satisfaction as she stepped off the scale.

Susan and Jean

Susan will never forget Jean's sixtieth birthday. What had started out as a festive occasion—mother and daughter meeting for lunch at a plush restaurant—suddenly turned into a nightmare.

As the maitre d' was leading them to their table, Susan watched in horror when her mother stumbled on the bottom step of the thickly carpeted stairway and fell.

It didn't seem to be a bad fall, but when Susan saw Jean's face turn ashen and heard her moan in pain, she knew it was serious. Later, in the hospital emergency room after the X-rays had been taken, Susan learned that her mother had fractured her left hip and surgery would be necessary.

After the operation, the surgeon talked with Susan in the waiting room. He tried to be reassuring about Jean's chances for recovery, but explained that the healing process would be slow, and that other fractures might occur later. He said that Jean's fall had probably not caused the fracture; instead, the fall was the result of a spontaneous fracture due to generalized osteoporosis, which made all Jean's bones, particularly the hip bones, extremely soft and weak.

Susan had read magazine articles about osteoporosis, but she had never thought her own mother would suffer from this disease.

What about Susan's bone health?

During her mother's recuperation, Susan was determined to find out more about osteoporosis and visited her physician. She learned that osteoporosis is a major cause of falls and fractures in older people, particularly women, and that medical complications from hip fractures are a leading cause of death in the elderly. Susan worries constantly about her mother. Although Jean has recovered and is walking again, she is often depressed about how her life has changed. Her fear of falling has turned her into a cautious, slow-moving woman who avoids many of the activities she used to enjoy.

Susan is also concerned about what may be happening to her own bones. Even though osteoporosis is usually diagnosed in older women, Susan has learned that it develops slowly through the lifespan and probably starts when women are in their thirties or even twenties. Moreover, Susan's doctor has told her that she fits the profile of a woman likely to develop osteoporosis.

Here's how Susan compares her own risk with the profile of a woman most at risk of developing osteoporosis.

WOMEN AT HIGH RISK MAY:	SUSAN'S RISK FACTORS:
Have family history of osteoporosis.	Her mother has osteoporosis.
Have ancestors from Britain, Europe, China, or Japan.	Grandparents came from Britain and northern Europe.
Have fair or thin skin.	Her skin is fair.
Be underweight.	She takes pride in her slim figure and diets frequently.
Have a slender build.	She is small-boned and petite.
Have had early menopause or removal of ovaries.	Neither condition applies to Susan.
Have poor eating habits: too much protein or sodium, not enough calcium.	Moderate protein intake; sodium high from canned and frozen foods; avoids dairy foods, especially when dieting.
Have had no children.	Susan has not had any children.
Never or rarely exercise.	Susan's tax consultant job keeps her at her desk most of the day, with little time or energy for regular exercise.
Have more than moderate amounts of: Caffeine	Susan drinks decaffeinated coffee and soft drinks without caffeine.
Alcohol	She sometimes has wine with dinner.
Cigarettes	She doesn't smoke.

17

Now that Susan recognizes her own susceptibility, she is firm in her resolve to take measures that will prevent her becoming another osteoporosis "statistic."

How Serious Is the Problem?

"Osteoporosis is a major public health problem that will only get worse as the population ages," stated Dr. William A. Peck, co-chairman of the 1987 Conference on Osteoporosis sponsored by the National Institutes of Health. Dr. Peck noted that medical and nursing home care for osteoporosis victims costs an estimated $7 billion to $10 billion, and that there is a mortality as high as 12 percent among hip fracture patients.

The conference participants supported recommendations of a previous NIH Consensus Conference on Osteoporosis: all adults should consume 1,000 milligrams of calcium a day, and postmenopausal women, particularly thin, white women, who are most at risk, should consume 1,500 milligrams a day.

The 1987 Conference concluded that the importance of calcium consumption is unquestioned, and affirmed that "well established" risk factors include the following:

1. Older age
2. Early menopause (either natural or from a hysterectomy)
3. Extreme immobility
4. Being a thin, white female

In addition, there is "moderate evidence," according to the 1987 Conference report, of other risk factors:

5. Low calcium intake
6. Cigarette smoking
7. Moderate alcohol consumption

Obviously, some of these risk factors are beyond your control. You can't halt the process of getting older; you can't change your race or gender; you can't alter the timing of natural menopause or change your body build. But you can add more calcium-rich foods to your daily diet to avoid the dilemma of the majority of American women whose intake of calcium falls below recommended levels.

On any given day, more than half the women in the United States have calcium intakes below the recommended level, and the proportion rises with age. *Between the ages of 18 and 30, when peak bone mass is developing, more than two-thirds of all U.S. females consume less than they need, and more than 75 percent of women over age 35 have insufficient calcium intake.*

These figures are alarming. They decisively demonstrate that American women are jeopardizing their bone health by not consuming enough calcium in their daily diets. In other words, most American women, like Susan, are likely candidates for osteoporosis.

There is also good news. Bone loss can be minimized or prevented by increased calcium intake. We have the power to help ourselves. Knowing that the calcium our bones need can be supplied by high calcium foods is certainly cause for optimism.

Looking Ahead

Laura and Jean, unfortunately, learned about osteoporosis only after they had already suffered its serious consequences. But they now understand that they can slow down the rate of bone loss by increasing their calcium intake.

Since Susan realizes her own susceptibility to bone fractures, she plans to be vigilant about calcium intake for the rest of her life. She knows that she has to begin while she is still young, to build up bone density in order to reduce the risk of osteoporosis after menopause.

With her doctor's help, she has chosen to change her dietary habits — to eat a normal balanced diet containing calcium-rich foods that will provide her with a wide variety of valuable nutrients — rather than having to depend on daily consumption of supplements and pills.

Susan and millions of other young women are keenly aware that their efforts to prevent osteoporosis need to begin at once. All of them can improve the odds against osteoporosis.

2
PRESCRIPTION FOR
BETTER BONE HEALTH

A FEW YEARS AGO most people had never heard of osteoporosis. They were probably aware that older people, especially women, seemed to break bones rather easily, but this was regarded as an inevitable part of aging rather than the result of years of inattention to bone health. Few people understood how or why the bones weaken with age.

Even now, after the considerable publicity directed at osteoporosis, it's hard for many of us to imagine that our bones are always changing or that bone building continues even after we've finished growing. There is certainly no outward evidence that any changes are taking place in the bones. They remain rigid; they always feel solid to the touch; they seem inert. We can witness other signs of getting older — a sprinkling of gray hair, a few wrinkles around the eyes. But we cannot see bone mass decreasing. We don't become aware that our bones have become weak and porous, fragile and brittle, until a fracture occurs.

The bones are the most dense organs in the body. Consisting primarily of calcium phosphate salts, bone tissue is continually being broken down and rebuilt throughout life under the influence of the body's hormones and the stresses imposed by muscle action.

Throughout infancy, childhood, and adolescence, the hormones promoting general growth predominate and the bones become longer, wider, and denser. At maturity, the bones do not get bigger, but their density may be altered by the flow of calcium into and out of them; the movement of calcium is, in turn, controlled by hormones and is closely related to the amount of calcium available. After the age of thirty-five to forty, many people do not absorb calcium as well as when they were younger, so *they need to consume even more calcium for the same benefit.*

The stresses of muscle and of gravity on bone, which also influences bone density, occurs with every movement we make, since every muscle is attached to the skeleton. Even the simple act of standing results in pulling action on the skeleton, as our body unconsciously resists gravity to maintain erect posture.

Importance of Calcium

Calcium is essential for many of the body's functions. It is needed to build bone tissue. Body cells and fluids need calcium for many life functions, particularly muscle (including heart) contraction and relaxation, activation of enzymes, stimulation of hormone secretion and action, blood coagulation, as well as integrity of substances holding cells together. These functions *take priority* over bone growth in the young. They also take priority over maintenance of bone strength in the adult; therefore, if there is not enough calcium in the diet, life continues, but bone slowly dissolves.

The density and, as a consequence, the strength of the bones depend on the amount of calcium available from the diet. Even a moderately low intake can have serious adverse effects. *If you are like many women who consume fewer than 500 milligrams of calcium each day, you may lose as much as 36 grams of calcium from your bones in the course of only one year to provide for the body's other needs.*

The amount of calcium in the total skeleton of an adult ranges between 1,000 and 1,300 grams for a man and between 775 and 950 grams for a woman (the variations depend on several factors, primarily height and genetic background). When about 30 percent of the calcium has been lost from a bone, it becomes osteoporotic and susceptible to fracture; this occurs at a loss of about 300 to 400 grams for a man and about 230 to 300 grams for a woman. *Therefore, if you were to lose 36 grams of calcium from your bones each year, it would take only from 6 to 12 years for osteoporosis to develop.*

About 98 percent of the calcium in a human is in the bones, about 1 percent is in the teeth, and the remaining 1 percent is dissolved in all the cells and fluids. The teeth are outside the metabolically active portion of the body and, once developed, cannot respond to the needs of the rest of the body. The calcium in the bones, however, moves back and forth, into and out of the body fluids as needed, under the control of the body's hormones.

Normal calcium loss

Calcium is depleted from the body normally and continuously. It is filtered from the blood by the kidneys, secreted in intestinal juices, and lost in small amounts in sweat, hair, and dead skin cells. For the average adult, these losses add up to approximately 300 milligrams per day, which must be replaced by the calcium in the diet.

Our bodies absorb different amounts of calcium at different times of our lives and under various dietary conditions. An average adult eating a balanced American diet, can absorb only about 35 percent of the calcium from the foods in that diet. An adult, therefore, must consume *at least* 800 milligrams of calcium a day just to offset the normal body loss of 300 milligrams, to avoid the gradual dissolving of bone tissues and to keep the calcium in the body fluids at the level necessary for all organs to function normally.

What is calcium balance?

When the amount of calcium absorbed from the diet is equal to that lost from the body, a state of balance is said to prevail. If the amount of calcium absorbed is greater than the losses, calcium goes into the bones and "positive balance" is present; if the losses are greater than the amount absorbed, calcium is leached from the bones and "negative balance" occurs. Positive balance is necessary for bone growth and repair. Negative balance results in demineralized bones, or osteoporosis.

To understand calcium balance, think of your bones as a "bank" for calcium. When you take in calcium from the foods you eat, it is deposited in your "bone bank." As long as you have a surplus of calcium deposited in the bone bank (that is, more calcium than is needed to keep the bones strong), you can continue to withdraw the calcium as needed for various body processes without harming your bones. If, however, your body's needs for calcium are consistently greater than the surplus calcium in the bone bank, then your withdrawals will mean that calcium is drawn out of the bones, producing a negative calcium balance.

A small negative calcium balance may not be serious in the short run. But if you allow it to continue for a sufficiently long period of time (30 to 40 years, for example), it will deplete so much calcium that the bones will be too weak to tolerate even a minor stress and will fracture.

Calcium Needs Throughout Life

The amount of calcium needed by the body depends on the stage of life.

Infancy

At birth, a 7-pound baby has about 30 grams of calcium in its bones. During the first two years of life, when growth is rapid, the requirement for calcium in the diet is very great proportional to body weight. A baby needs about 360 milligrams of calcium per day (about 20 milligrams per pound) for the first six months and about 540 milligrams per day for the next year. Since milk is the primary component of the diet during infancy, this amount is easily provided.

Childhood

During childhood (from about eighteen months of age to ten years), growth continues, but at a slower rate and the proportional requirement drops to about 10 milligrams per pound per day. About 800 milligrams of calcium per day is adequate to meet this need.

Adolescence

During adolescence, the growth rate increases rapidly, and the total calcium requirement rises to about 1,200 to 1,400 milligrams per day. If sufficient bone mass is not built up, the teen may become at risk for osteoporosis in later years when the body's ability to absorb calcium is reduced. Surveys by the U.S. Department of Agriculture reveal that adolescent males are protecting their bones much more effectively than adolescent females because they consume about 30 percent more calcium than adolescent females. Young women, concerned about staying slim, often restrict food intake quite severely, thus decreasing their intake of calcium as well as other nutrients.

Adults

When the growth spurt is over and maturity is reached, the minimum requirement drops to about 800 milligrams per day. With aging, changes in hormones and in the efficiency of absorption from the intestines increase the requirements for calcium again, to levels of about 1,200 to

1,400 milligrams per day for post-menopausal women taking estrogen and for men over age sixty. Post-menopausal women who are not taking estrogen need even more—up to 1,500 or 2,000 milligrams of calcium per day.

Pregnancy and lactation

Even though there is some evidence that the efficiency of calcium absorption increases temporarily during pregnancy, the addition of at least 400 milligrams of calcium per day is recommended because there is a possible link between calcium loss during pregnancy and lactation, and later development of osteoporosis.

During the last trimester of pregnancy, 25 to 35 grams of calcium are deposited in the fetal skeleton. This amount of calcium is withdrawn from the mother's body at the rate of about 10 grams per month.

Think about those figures for a few moments. Remember that one gram equals 1,000 milligrams. Therefore, 10 grams of calcium equals 10,000 milligrams. If you divide 10,000 milligrams by 30 days (1 month), you will see that *every day* during the last three months of pregnancy, approximately 333 milligrams of calcium are deposited in the fetal skeleton. During lactation, 500 to 700 milligrams of calcium per day may be secreted in milk.

That calcium, which is necessary to maintain bone growth in the fetus and the nursing infant, has to come from somewhere. *If the calcium is not available to the fetus and infant from the mother's dietary sources, then the calcium is withdrawn from the mother's bones.*

Why We're Not Getting Enough Calcium

Few women realize the vital importance of adequate calcium intake. Young women may think about the effects of what they eat on their figure, or their skin, or, perhaps, on their energy level. But the possibility of developing weak bones seems remote indeed. It is difficult to make the connection between today's diet and a broken hip twenty to forty years in the future. Other factors, as well, may account for the widespread calcium deficiency among American women.

"Milk drinking is for kids"

Contrary to popular opinion, the need for calcium increases as people grow older. Yet, for most of us, our calcium intake was probably higher when we were younger.

Many of us received dire warnings from our parents that we would stop growing properly if we didn't finish every drop of milk in our glass. Some mothers made their messages stronger by not serving dessert until the glass was empty. Though we grumbled, we swallowed the milk along with the idea that we needed it for "strong bones and teeth." We accepted the message as long as we had proof that our body was still growing.

But once we became full-grown — once our dress or suit size stayed the same year after year — most of us figured that our bones and teeth must have enough calcium to last us forever. We made the dietary passage into adulthood by freeing ourselves from parental admonitions. We pushed away the glass of milk and exchanged it for the badge of adulthood: a cup of steaming hot coffee or a can of cola.

We were concerned that business associates at the restaurant lunch table might raise their eyebrows if we ordered a glass of milk. The only time it became acceptable for women to become "public" milk drinkers was during pregnancy and lactation, when they conscientiously drank milk "for the sake of the baby." Few understood, and few doctors explained, that it was not only the health of the baby that was at stake, but that a woman's bones would later pay the price when calcium intake was not sufficient.

Fear that dairy products are fattening

Some pharmaceutical companies would like us to believe that it's impossible to get enough calcium from food without gaining weight.

A recent advertisement for calcium supplements splashed across the pages of women's magazines boasted that the manufacturer's product "contains more calcium than a half-quart of milk — *without the calories.*" Another manufacturer distributes a booklet to physicians that states: "Even a well-balanced diet cannot provide enough calcium every day *without also giving excess calories.*"

Such advertising fosters the myth that dairy products make us gain weight. Yet most nutritionists agree that excess calories can usually be traced to the "fats and sweets" category: high calorie foods that dieters often forget to count, like the glazed doughnuts passed around at office meetings.

It's time to set the record straight. Dairy products are now available in such a wide array of choices that even the most rigid dieters can get a major portion of their daily calcium from skim milk, nonfat or low fat yogurt, and part-skim cheese. These low fat dairy products contain the same amount of calcium as the whole-milk versions, with fewer calories and less fat. We can't, of course, expect to avoid gaining a few pounds if we rely on ice cream as our sole source of calcium. But we can certainly maintain a moderate calorie level with a nutritious combination of nonfat and low fat dairy products and other high calcium foods.

Soft drinks intake up; milk down

Forbes magazine recently reported that the soft drink industry made the highest profits of any business in the United States during the previous five-year period. The latest figures from the U.S. Department of Agriculture confirm that Americans are drinking soft drinks at an unprecedented rate.

There are more alarming facts revealed by the U.S. Department of Agriculture, which compared the average one-day soft drink consumption of 19- to 34-year-old females in two different years: 1977 and 1985. Researchers found an increase of more than 34 percent in soft drink consumption, while milk intake dropped almost 9 percent during that same time. This inverse relationship between the consumption of soft drinks and milk may be a significant factor in the rise in osteoporosis in the United States in recent years.

Here is serious cause for concern. Women in the age group studied are the ones who should be taking the best care of their bones to prevent osteoporosis in later years. Yet, during these critical years, too many women are reaching into their refrigerators for a soda can rather than a milk carton.

Ads for diet drinks make it tempting to give up milk. A beverage that promises a sweet taste and the ability to make us "feel full" without calories has an irresistible appeal, and the soft drink industry has successfully sold these products as the easy road to slim figures.

The newer soft drink products are promoted to appeal to health-conscious Americans because they are sugar-free and often caffeine-free. They are also nutrient-free. They provide no nutritional benefits at all, and the cola-flavored varieties may even have an adverse affect on calcium absorption.

Dieting

The lure of losing weight in "14 days or your money back" is almost irresistible. You may get your money back, but it will be more difficult to restore the density of your bones once bone mass is lost. Diets that ignore sound nutritional principles may lead to eventual bone loss if foods that are good sources of calcium are avoided. Furthermore, "crash dieting" with an intake of less than 800 calories per day is likely to result in calcium being *pulled out of the bones*.

Adolescent women, especially, are in greatest jeopardy for later osteoporosis because they are not consuming enough calcium during the years when they are building bones. They believe the myth that only the gaunt get their man, and they follow drastic reducing diets. But both male and female adolescents should be consuming from 200 to 400 milligrams of calcium *above* the U.S. RDA of 1,000 milligrams.

Some young women who become victims of the eating disorders *anorexia* or *bulimia* develop osteoporosis decades earlier than other women. The self-imposed starvation and/or vomiting lead to very low intakes of dietary calcium and other nutrients necessary for bone strength at ages when the requirements are highest. Moreover, the extreme weight loss that occurs results in cessation of estrogen production — in effect, very early menopause. These young women often have pathological bone fractures in their teens or early twenties as a result of starvation and the obsessive exercise programs they impose on themselves.

Thinking it's too late

If you are past menopause, don't throw up your hands in despair and think there's no chance of improving your bone health. No matter what your age, it is *never* too late, because you *can* slow down the process that leads to weakened bones.

Many research studies have revealed that age-related bone loss may be slowed down by increased calcium consumption. However, since aging does decrease the body's ability to absorb calcium, mature people need to learn how much calcium their bodies actually require and choose foods that will fulfill that requirement. *Even if your bones have already lost enough calcium to become osteoporotic, there is much you can do to prevent further loss of bone and the possibility of fractures.*

How Much Calcium Is Enough?

Public health, medical, and nutrition experts have no simple answer for the woman who wants to know how much calcium she should be consuming every day. There are two sets of suggested recommendations for daily calcium intake —each from a different, but equally authoritative source.

One is called the "Recommended Dietary Allowances," abbreviated RDA, and the other is called the "U.S. Recommended Daily Allowances," and is abbreviated U.S. RDA. The words are similar, but the amounts recommended for daily intake of nutrients may be different. The following information should help clear up some of the confusion.

RDA (Recommended Dietary Allowances)

These are nutritional recommendations made by the Food and Nutrition Board of the National Research Council of the National Academy of Sciences in Washington, DC. They are intended as guidelines for population groups rather than individuals, and cover the amount of protein, along with 19 vitamins and minerals, that are recommended for "healthy" populations. Revised at approximately five-year intervals, the recommendations were most recently issued in 1980. The anticipated 1985 revisions were postponed, but there are indications that the majority of experts are recommending increases in calcium intake for both adults and older women.

POPULATION GROUP	RDA for CALCIUM (mg)
Birth - 6 months	360
6 months - 1 year	540
1 year - 10 years	800
11 years - 18 years	1,200
Adults	800
Pregnant and lactating women	1,200

U.S. RDA (U.S. Recommended Daily Allowances)

The cereal box that you gaze at with sleepy eyes at the breakfast table proclaims in large letters that a serving provides "100% of the daily requirements of vitamins and minerals." These requirements are determined by the U.S. Food and Drug Administration, which sets the dietary standards on which the nutritional labeling of food products is based.

Many food packages carry listings titled "Nutrition Information per Serving" and "Percentage of U.S. Recommended Daily Allowances (U.S. RDA)." The percentages are given for eight nutrients including calcium. The U.S. RDA is issued for four different population groups, as follows:

POPULATION GROUP	U.S. RDA for CALCIUM (mg)
Children under 1 year	600
Children 1 - 4 years	800
Children over 4 - adults	1,000
Pregnant and lactating women	1,300

What is a confused health consumer to do?

As you can see, the RDA figures are slightly lower than those of the U.S. RDA. Many health and nutrition experts have been urging the Food and Nutrition Board to raise the RDA for calcium, and the Board is expected to do so.

The panel of experts at the NIH conference on osteoporosis stated that "the RDA for calcium (at 800 milligrams) is evidently too low, particularly for post-menopausal women, and may well be too low for elderly men." They cited evidence that post-menopausal women who are not treated with estrogen require about 1,500 milligrams of calcium daily to maintain calcium balance. *"It seems likely," the report concludes, "that an increase in calcium intake to 1,000 to 1,500 milligrams a day, beginning well before menopause, will reduce the incidence of osteoporosis in post-menopausal women."*

The guideline for calcium intake for food labeling is based on the "general population" category (children over 4 - adults) of the U.S. RDA, and is 1,000 milligrams. For example, on a milk carton, a serving (8 oz) of milk is listed as containing 30% of the U.S. RDA for calcium.

Since the U.S. RDA guidelines were first established, medical and nutritional research has revealed that calcium needs may vary considerably for different population and gender groups. We have, therefore, prepared our own recommendations for daily intake of calcium for men and women in fifteen different categories.

Use the following chart to find your appropriate age/gender group and you can determine what your daily calcium needs are. The intake recommendations are listed both in milligrams and in percentages of the U.S. RDA for each population group.

You should always consult with your own physician about the calcium intake level that best meets your individual health needs.

IF YOU ARE IN THIS POPULATION GROUP	YOU SHOULD BE CONSUMING THIS AMOUNT OF CALCIUM (mg)	EQUIVALENT U.S. RDA
Birth - 6 months	360	60%
6 months - 1 year	540	90%
1 year - 18 months	540	68%
18 months - 4 years	800	100%
4 years - 10 years	800	80%
10 years - 18 years	1,200 - 1,400	120% -140%
Pregnant adolescent women	1,600 - 1,800	125% -140%
Pregnant women over 18	1,600	125%
Lactating women	1,600	125%
Women, 18 - menopause	1,000 - 1,200	100% -120%
Post-menopausal women, not taking estrogen	1,500 - 2,000	150% -200%
Post-menopausal women, taking estrogen	1,200 - 1,400	120% -140%
Men 18 - 45	1,000 - 1,200	100% -120%
Men 45 - 60	1,000 - 1,200	100% -120%
Men over 60	1,200 - 1,400	120% -140%

After you and your physician have determined your individual calcium needs, use the listings in the Calcium and Calorie Counter to select daily food choices that add up to the percentage appropriate for your age/gender group.

3

INFLUENCES ON CALCIUM ABSORPTION AND RETENTION

ALTHOUGH CALCIUM IS the body's most plentiful mineral, it must be consumed daily and it must be absorbed by the body, to prevent the bones from eventually becoming demineralized. The absorption and retention of calcium by the body is influenced not only by the amount of calcium consumed, but also by many other factors, including the amounts of other nutrients in the diet, the amount of exercise done, and the level of the body's secretion of various hormones.

Hormones

Estrogen

Estrogen is involved in bone production and has a protective influence on bone loss. The usual slow decrease in bone calcium content, which starts at about age thirty-five to forty in both men and women, accelerates in women whose estrogen level has decreased, either because they have had their ovaries removed surgically or have undergone a natural menopause. The rate of loss can be slowed down by replacing the estrogen. Although estrogen alone cannot reverse the loss of calcium from the bones, when used in adequate dosage along with adequate amounts of calcium in the diet, it does slow (or even stop) the process started by the absence of the female hormones.

According to the NIH conference report, estrogen (along with calcium) is "the mainstay of prevention and management of osteoporosis. A substantial reduction in hip or wrist fractures resulted in women whose estrogen replacement was begun within a few years of menopause. Even when started as late as six years after the menopause, estrogen may prevent further loss of bone mass, but does not restore it to pre-

33

menopausal levels." For women well past the menopause, however, the report states that "there is no convincing evidence that initiating estrogen therapy in elderly women will prevent osteoporosis."

Most physicians recommend that when estrogen is taken, appropriate amounts of progesterone be taken as well, in order to avoid possible problems such as malignancies or cysts.

The decision concerning the initiation of estrogen therapy is made by the physician with the patient, after a thorough examination of the patient's medical history and full consideration of the consequences of such therapy. How long estrogen should be taken has not yet been determined. Some studies show that when estrogen is discontinued, even after five years, bone loss accelerates again.

It should be emphasized that the taking of estrogens by a woman who still is having normal menstrual cycles will not prevent osteoporosis. Increased bone loss may occur following the decline of normal estrogen supply, whether this is the result of biological menopause or surgical removal of the ovaries. When estrogen production decreases, treatment with these hormones may minimize the bone loss. Before menopause, loss of bone leading to osteoporosis is due to other factors which we will discuss later.

Other hormones

Parathyroid and *calcitonin* are the principal hormones that act together with vitamin D to control the formation and breakdown of bones, the absorption of calcium from the diet, and the losses of calcium from the body.

Parathyroid hormone is produced by the parathyroid glands, which are located near the thyroid. Parathyroid hormone is "turned on" by low calcium levels or high phosphorus levels in the blood. Even though the parathyroid hormone increases the absorption of calcium from the diet and decreases the loss of calcium in the urine, it increases the amount of calcium removed from the bones. Overactivity of parathyroid hormone, therefore, increases bone loss by reducing bone calcium.

Calcitonin, which is produced by cells in the parathyroid and thyroid glands, functions directly opposite to the parathyroid hormone. Calcitonin lowers the amount of calcium in the blood and tissue fluids by increasing the deposition of calcium into the bones. Calcitonin is released when blood levels of calcium increase or levels of phosphorus drop.

The "push-pull" effects of parathyroid and calcitonin hormones help to keep the blood calcium concentration normal and, when there is enough calcium in the diet, to keep the bone calcium normal.

Many other hormones also affect calcium movement into and out of the bones and body. Excessive amounts of *thyroid* hormone increase the breakdown of bone and loss of calcium by the intestine and the kidney. *Cortisone,* whether taken as a medication or produced by the body, increases calcium losses and slows down bone formation. In diabetes, the lack of *insulin* may also affect the bones by causing increased loss of calcium from the body and preventing normal new bone growth.

It is obvious that the body's hormones may influence the development of osteoporosis by increasing the losses of calcium from the body, by preventing proper absorption of calcium from the diet, by increasing bone breakdown, or by preventing bone formation. Losses of calcium from the bones and the body ("negative calcium balance") result from overactivity of the parathyroid hormone, thyroid hormone or cortisone, and from deficiencies of estrogen or insulin. Correction of such abnormalities may prevent or slow down the development of osteoporosis. Similarly, with some individuals, giving additional calcitonin (along with calcium) may counteract some of the harmful effects of the other hormone imbalances. This determination can only be made by your physician.

Exercise

An appropriate amount of physical activity, too, is essential for maintenance of bone calcium. Immobilization removes the stress stimuli (gravity and muscle action) necessary for incorporation of calcium into new bone. Thus, people of any age who are at complete bed rest after serious injury, heart attack, or stroke start losing calcium from their bones within the first twenty-four hours and continue to lose it rapidly until they start moving about again.

Similarly, astronauts lose calcium from the moment they enter zero gravity conditions and continue to lose while in orbit, even though they may be exercising their muscles actively or isometrically. As soon as the astronauts return to normal gravity they start retaining calcium again. This suggests that the effect of exercise on bones is due to resisting gravity, and explains why "weight-bearing" exercises (walking, running, bicycling, tennis, etc.) that resist gravity are better for bone building than such exercises as swimming or "lying down" mat exercises.

The data are still inconclusive as to just how much exercise is required to prevent calcium losses, and whether or not increasing the amount of exercise produces better calcium retention. It is generally agreed, however, that any physical activity, no matter how mild, is better than none at all.

Since many people who already have osteoporosis have had painful fractures of the spine, hip, or arms, they may need pain medication, braces, and medical supervision of planned physical activity to promote healing and prevent further bone destruction. The evidence available suggests that even a mild exercise such as regular daily walking is helpful in stimulating bone repair and growth. If you have had fractures or if you develop pain with activity, check with your physician before exercising.

Excessive exercise, on the other hand, may be conducive to early development of osteoporosis. Many women professional athletes have trained to the point of stopping their menstrual cycles; they have been found to develop osteoporosis at younger ages and of greater severity than non-athletes.

Dietary Influences

Many components of the diet influence the absorption and retention of calcium. Some have a positive influence; others may increase the dietary requirement for calcium.

Vitamin D

Vitamin D is needed for the absorption of calcium from the intestines and for the incorporation of calcium into bone. The U.S. RDA for vitamin D is 400 International Units (IU) per day. With aging in some individuals, the conversion of vitamin D to its hormonally active form by the liver and kidneys may be decreased and thus the requirement for vitamin D may be increased.

Large excesses of vitamin D — greater than 1,000 IU per day — can destroy bone. Some individuals, however, because of underlying diseases such as liver, kidney, or malabsorption syndromes may require high doses of vitamin D. These should be used only under close medical supervision.

Vitamin D is made normally by the body through the action of certain wavelengths of ultraviolet light, derived primarily from sunlight, on cholesterol in the skin. (Fluorescent lights of the "daylight" type also emit ultraviolet rays of the same wavelength as sunlight.) Vitamin D may also be obtained from the diet, primarily from milk. Most milk has vitamin D added to provide 400 IU per quart.

Vitamin D deficiency in adults usually produces a condition known as osteomalacia or "adult rickets." In this disorder, there is an abnormal supporting structure for the bone mineral, which does not take up calcium. As a result, bones are very soft and may fracture, just as in osteoporosis. Commonly, patients with bone diseases as a result of inadequate nutrition have a combination of osteomalacia and osteoporosis.

Lactose

Lactose, the natural sugar found in milk (which does not taste sweet), appears to improve the absorption of calcium, particularly in infants. Many individuals, however, suffer from a condition known as lactose intolerance; they have a genetically programmed loss of the intestinal enzyme *lactase*, which normally digests the lactose present in milk. As a result, they may develop abdominal discomfort, gas, and diarrhea after ingesting large amounts of lactose. Although this is uncomfortable, it does not lead to nutritional deficiencies.

Lactose intolerance is a fairly common problem that affects non-Caucasians at a higher rate (3 out of 10) than Caucasians (1 out of 10). If you are lactose intolerant, you should avoid large amounts of soft cheeses such as Brie, Camembert, cream cheese, and neufchatel, and you may have difficulty with foods containing nonfat instant dry milk or evaporated milk.

Don't jeopardize your bone health by avoiding all dairy products, because such drastic measures are usually not necessary. You can probably eat "hard" cheeses such as Cheddar and Swiss, which have had the lactose largely removed in the cheesemaking process, when the whey is drained. And don't overlook yogurt, which is one of the best sources of calcium. If you purchase a brand that contains "active yogurt cultures," the healthful bacteria present in this type of yogurt work in the intestine to digest the lactose that may be present from other foods.

Many lactose intolerant people may find they can eat yogurt cream cheese, a tasty replacement for commercial cream cheese that can be easily made by draining the whey from plain low fat or nonfat yogurt.

37

Only about half the lactose contained in the yogurt remains in the yogurt cream cheese. Instructions for making yogurt cream cheese are in Chapter 8, and suggestions for using it, and recipes, are in Chapter 10.

For those who are lactose intolerant, LactAid milk, a lactose-reduced milk (1% fat), is available in the dairy cases of supermarkets in many parts of the country in quart cartons. An 8-ounce serving of milk in the blue LactAid carton contains 30 percent of the U.S. RDA for calcium; 8 ounces of milk in the red "Calcimilk" carton is 50 percent of the U.S. RDA. LactAid cheese slices are also available.

To determine the availability of LactAid products in your area, call 1-800-257-8650. LactAid and other commercial enzyme products, which are available at drug stores, can convert the lactose in regular milk into easily digestible sugars. These preparations may be added to milk or taken by mouth as tablets along with milk.

Oxalates and phytates

Oxalates. Many foods of plant origin have oxalates (oxalic acid) in them, which form an insoluble substance in the digestive tract that prevents calcium from being absorbed. Their effects may be made worse by other substances, such as vitamin C, which are changed to oxalates in the body. Oxalates also increase the tendency to kidney stones in some people.

The United States Department of Agriculture's latest (1984) edition of Handbook 8-11, *Composition of Foods: Vegetables and Vegetable Products*, includes the following information about oxalic acid:

> Oxalic acid can combine with calcium and magnesium to form highly insoluble compounds which can make these minerals unavailable to the body. However, *most foods do not contain enough oxalic acid to combine with a significant amount of calcium or magnesium from the same food or from another source.*
>
> Those foods that contain high amounts of oxalic acid usually contain sufficient calcium or magnesium to bind with all the oxalic acid in that food. Therefore, *oxalic acid in these foods would not interfere with the calcium and magnesium availability of other foods in the diet.*

Some consumers who are concerned about osteoporosis have refrained from buying greens, spinach, and other vegetables because they have read that oxalic acid may interfere with calcium absorption. Except for raw spinach in salads, most foods with oxalic acid are served cooked and eaten in small quantities. Cooking largely destroys oxalic acid, as does adding vinegar or lemon juice when cooking. Unless you consume large amounts of raw spinach, Swiss chard, and beet greens every day, it is not likely that oxalic acid will have a major effect on your absorption of calcium from other foods.

OXALIC ACID CONTENT OF SELECTED VEGETABLES

VEGETABLE	GRAMS OXALIC ACID PER 100 GRAMS (3.5 oz)	VEGETABLE	GRAMS OXALIC ACID PER 100 GRAMS (3.5 oz)
Amaranth	1.09	Lettuce	.33
Asparagus	.13	Okra	.05
Beans, snap	.36	Onion	.05
Beet greens	.61	Parsley	1.70
Broccoli	.19	Peas	.05
Brussels sprouts	.36	Peppers	.04
Cabbage	.10	Potatoes	.05
Carrots	.50	Radish	.48
Cauliflower	.15	Rutabaga	.03
Celery	.19	Spinach	.97
Chives	1.48	Squash	.02
Collards	.45	Sweet potatoes	.24
Corn, sweet	.01	Tomatoes	.05
Cucumbers	.02	Turnips	.21
Eggplant	.19	Turnip greens	.05
Endive	.11	Watercress	.31
Kale	.02		

Source: Agriculture Handbook 8-11, U.S. Department of Agriculture, Human Nutrition Service, "Composition of Foods: Vegetables and Vegetable Products," revised August, 1984, Washington, D.C.

Phytates. Whole grains and other high fiber foods contain large amounts of phytates, which combine with calcium to produce a substance that cannot be absorbed by the intestines. Phytates only become an important factor in the diet when foods containing them are eaten in large amounts and calcium intake is low.

As with oxalates, if calcium intake is liberal from other sources, phytates shouldn't have a significant effect on calcium absorption.

Protein

The average American diet provides about 100 to 120 grams of protein daily, which offers an adequate safety buffer for the average requirement of about 70 grams per day. Diets very high in animal protein, however, increase loss of calcium in the urine, thereby increasing the need for dietary calcium. Intakes greater than 180 to 200 grams per day become important in terms of calcium loss; this would be seen in the individual who eats a pound or more of meat per day.

Sodium

Sodium is excreted by the kidneys and pulls calcium out of the body with it. In general, the more sodium that is consumed, the more that is excreted and, therefore, the more calcium that is lost. This may be a small but significant and steady loss in people whose diets are habitually high in salt content.

Most people are unaware that sodium has a negative effect on their calcium balance. If you want to reduce your sodium intake, you should be aware of some facts:

Processed meats are very high in sodium. A single hot dog, for example, contains more sodium than four glasses of milk, or three 8-ounce containers of yogurt, or six slices of natural Swiss cheese.

Natural Swiss contains less sodium than any other hard cheese, and it contains about one-fourth as much sodium as processed Swiss.

One tablespoon of bottled Italian salad dressing contains more than twice as much sodium as a glass of milk.

Eight ounces of canned mushroom soup contains about five times more sodium than 8 ounces of yogurt.

Phosphorus

Phosphorus, which is normally bound to the calcium in the bones, is an essential component of bone. Nevertheless, excesses of phosphorus can prevent adequate absorption of calcium. In young infants, the ratio is extremely critical and an excessive intake of phosphorus can prevent normal bone growth. Adults have much more tolerance.

Since phosphorus is present in virtually all foods, deficiencies are rare except in some disease conditions or when certain medications are taken. Excesses of phosphorus, on the other hand, are very common, particularly in the American diet. Phosphorus is present in grains, milk, meats, and eggs. Cola drinks contain an especially large amount. Only milk has enough calcium to balance the phosphorus in it. If large amounts of meat, grains, or cola-type soft drinks are consumed, the ratio of phosphorus to calcium in the diet may become too high.

Magnesium

Magnesium is one of the major minerals in the diet. There have been studies that suggest that many Americans do not get enough magnesium in their usual foods. In magnesium-deficient animals, parathyroid hormone action is abnormal and calcium absorption is decreased. However, excesses of magnesium may also be harmful in preventing normal absorption of calcium. There is no evidence that magnesium deficiency is a problem in humans. Magnesium is found primarily in green vegetables.

Other trace minerals and vitamins

Many other trace minerals and vitamins are present in the diet and in bones. Animal research has shown that deficiencies of some of these may prevent normal bone metabolism and contribute to the development of osteoporosis. These include the minerals boron and zinc, and vitamins K and C. However, excesses of these, particularly zinc and vitamin C (as well as excesses of other minerals and vitamins such as aluminum, molybdenum, and vitamin A) may actually produce osteoporosis. At this time there is no evidence for recommended addition of any of these to treat osteoporosis.

Fluoride

The fluoride in drinking water is incorporated into the bones along with calcium and makes them more resistant to bone loss. People who live in areas where the water supply is deficient in fluoride have more osteoporosis than those who use water with a natural fluoride content or where the water is fluoridated (to a level of one part per million).

Much higher doses of fluoride have been given as medication to slow

41

the breakdown of bone in osteoporosis and thus increase the density; however, when fluoride is consumed for several years in these high doses, it can cause the bones to become abnormal in other respects and become susceptible to fractures.

Fat

The amount and kind of fat in the diet may have a slight effect on the absorption of calcium, particularly in people who have a problem with intestinal malabsorption of fat. When fat is poorly absorbed, dietary vitamin D cannot be absorbed either. If the fat is saturated (such as animal fat, coconut oil, and cottonseed oil), the unabsorbed fat forms insoluble (and unabsorbable) complexes with calcium (called "calcium soaps").

Caffeine

Caffeine increases the excretion of calcium through the urine. If you take several coffee breaks during the day, and perhaps drink a few colas too, your caffeine intake may exceed the 1,000 milligram-per-day level that may begin to affect your body's retention of calcium. It is estimated that the average daily per capita intake of caffeine in the U.S. is about 200 milligrams.

Coffee is the most common source of caffeine in the American diet, with about 90 percent of our caffeine intake coming from coffee. The caffeine in coffee is variable, and depends on the amount of caffeine in the coffee beans and the method of preparation. The Food and Drug Administration estimates about 115 milligrams of caffeine in a 5-ounce cup of coffee brewed by drip method, 80 milligrams when brewed in a percolator, and 65 milligrams for instant coffee.

Tea drinkers may find it equally difficult to assess the amount of caffeine they're pouring from their teapots, but they usually consume less caffeine per cup: 40 milligrams for a major U.S. brand of tea; 60 milligrams for an imported brand.

Soft drinks. A recent report of the Federal Drug Administration revealed that the caffeine in cola-type and other soft drinks accounts for 80 to 90 percent of the estimated two million pounds of caffeine *added* to foods annually in the U.S.

Following is the caffeine content in some popular soft drinks:

SOFT DRINK	CAFFEINE / 6 FL OZ
Coca-Cola Classic/Diet Coke	23 mg
Dr. Pepper	26 mg
Mello Yellow	26 mg
Mountain Dew	27 mg
Mr. Pibb	20 mg
Pepsi-Cola	19 mg
Pepsi, Diet	18 mg
Tab	23 mg

Caffeine also is an ingredient in chocolate and in many over-the-counter headache, cold, and weight-loss pills.

Alcohol

Alcohol may be a significant factor in bone loss when consumed chronically and in large amounts. If you drink a glass of wine with dinner or have an occasional cocktail, you probably don't need to be terribly concerned. But if you drink regularly, even just as a "social drinker," you should be aware that alcohol may increase the risk of osteoporosis.

Alcohol affects the body's metabolism of vitamin D. After alcohol is absorbed and broken down in the liver, it interferes with the activation of vitamin D (activated vitamin D helps the absorption of calcium). It may also lead to liver damage, again preventing the conversion of vitamin D to its active form. Even in moderate amounts, alcohol may indirectly affect bone loss by decreasing the appetite so that the consumption of calcium-rich foods is lowered.

Research studies on men, who are about six times less likely than women to develop osteoporosis, have suggested a link between alcohol consumption and osteoporosis. High consumers of alcohol have about two and a half times the incidence of osteoporosis than a comparable group of non-drinkers. As we noted in our discussion of vitamin D, chronic alcoholics are more prone to vitamin D deficiency osteomalacia (poorly mineralized bone) as well.

Medications and drugs

Some *diuretics*, such as furosemide (Lasix) produce urinary losses of calcium. The *thiazides*, on the other hand, may lead to the retention of calcium. *Anyone whose physician has prescribed a thiazide diuretic should not take a calcium supplement without that physician's approval*, because blood calcium levels may become very high.

Aluminum-containing *antacids* (such as Di-Gel, Gaviscon, Gelusil, Maalox, Mylanta, Rolaids, and Tempo), by preventing absorption of phosphate, increase bone breakdown and increase urinary loss of calcium. *Isoniazid (INH)*, used in the treatment of tuberculosis, increases calcium loss. *Anticoagulants*, particularly heparin, prevent calcium from being deposited into bone and thus increase loss.

Antibiotics of the tetracycline family bind calcium in the intestine; while this is insignificant for calcium balance, it prevents the antibiotic from being effective. *Anyone who is taking a tetracycline should not drink milk or take a calcium supplement within two hours (before or after) the antibiotic.*

Listed below are the names of drugs in the tetracycline "family":

TRADE NAME	TETRACYCLINE
Achromycin	tetracycline
Azotrex	tetracycline
Declomycin	demeclocycline
Doxycycline	doxycycline
Minocin	minocycline
Mysteclin	tetracycline
Oxymycin	oxytetracycline
Panmycin	tetracycline
Robitet	tetracycline
Rondomycin	methacycline
Sumycin	tetracycline
Terra-Cortril	oxytetracycline
Terramycin	oxytetracycline
Tetracycline	tetracycline
Tetracyn	tetracycline
Tetrastatin	tetracycline
Tetrex	tetracycline
Topicycline	tetracycline
Urobiotic	oxytetracycline
Vibramycin	doxycycline

Nicotine

Cigarette smoking may increase the risk of bone loss. Nicotine from tobacco increases calcium losses, probably by action on the kidney. The research studies on alcoholics mentioned earlier noted the following: (a) that the risk of spinal osteoporosis was significantly greater among men who smoked than those who did not, and (b) the risk was even greater for those who both smoked and drank alcohol to excess than those who only smoked or only drank.

Smoking may lower estrogen levels, either directly or because of its effect on body fat, and is therefore linked to earlier menopause and increased incidence of osteoporosis. Thus smokers have increased risks, not only of heart disease, emphysema, and cancer, but of painful osteoporotic fractures as well.

Drugs in the future

Researchers are studying many new drugs and medications for the prevention and treatment of osteoporosis. Most are still being evaluated in animals only, but one class of compounds is beginning to show great promise in patients with osteoporosis. These are called *diphosphonates*.

Diphosphonates have been used in the past in the treatment of other disorders of bone metabolism and in recent studies have been given to patients with osteoporosis, with good results at present. They are being given in pill form for several weeks of each year along with continuous high intakes of calcium in the diet. These substances are incorporated into the bones along with calcium and make the bone more resistant to breakdown.

Summing Up

A complex interaction of hormone metabolism and diet affects the movement of calcium within and out of the bones and body. When this process results in increasing bone formation, it produces a positive calcium balance. When it results in increased bone breakdown, it causes negative calcium balance.

The key to the final outcome is the amount of calcium in the diet. The following factors influence the absorption and losses of calcium consumed with the diet, either as food or supplements: (a) hormones such as parathyroid hormone, calcitonin, estrogens, thyroid hormone, or insulin; (b) dietary substances such as vitamin D, phosphorus, protein; (c) drugs such as fluoride, alcohol, or diphosphonates.

4
ASK THE DOCTOR

FOLLOWING ARE some of the questions asked most frequently by patients concerned with problems of osteoporosis.

Q. I am 40 years old, and have increased my intake of calcium to avoid getting osteoporosis the way my mother did. My husband, who is 45, says he doesn't need to eat more calcium-containing foods because osteoporosis is a disease only women get. Is that true?

A. Not true at all. It is true that at any age, more women have osteoporosis than do men. It is also true that women usually develop osteoporosis at an earlier age than do men. However, men are also at risk.

There are more women than men with osteoporosis for several reasons. Men continue to increase the size and calcium content of their bones until about age 21 to 25, whereas women reach puberty and end puberty at earlier ages, with maximum skeletal maturity at about age 16 to 18. Thus women at adulthood usually have less calcium within their bones than do men. The normal decrease in bone calcium content starts about 20 to 25 years after maturity and therefore is apparent in women at about age 40 and in men about five to ten years later. Furthermore, the decline in estrogens in women at menopause may increase the rate of calcium loss from the bones. As a result, we see osteoporosis with fractures in women most commonly at about ages 50 to 55; in men, this doesn't occur until almost 65 to 70. As more men live longer we may expect to find even more osteoporosis in men, although at a later age than in women.

Q. I am 49 years old and have not been a milk drinker. I fit the pattern of the woman who develops osteoporosis. My menstrual periods have become irregular in the past six months. How would I

know if I am developing osteoporosis? Is there a blood test or any other kind of test I could take or do I have to wait until I fracture my spine or hip?

A. If you believe you fall in the group of those who may develop osteoporosis, it is not too late to change your life style now. Increase your intake of calcium, cut back on meals high in salt and meat, give up cola beverages, start a regular program of exercise, and see your doctor for the possibility of starting to take estrogen (and progesterone) supplements now.

Blood tests cannot predict or diagnose osteoporosis; the blood content of calcium stays normal at the expense of the bones unless you have some other disorder. Routine X-rays may show osteoporosis before fractures occur, but by the time the radiologist can detect loss of bone mineral on a standard X-ray, at least 30 percent of the mineral has already been lost. A more sensitive technique, bone densitometry, is available at many centers specializing in the treatment of osteoporosis. A low value on a single occasion may suggest osteoporosis but does not confirm the diagnosis since there are errors of over- and under-diagnosis by this procedure as with others. Although the equipment for bone densitometry is becoming more widely available, most osteoporosis experts believe its diagnostic value is not great, but that it may be of help in following the progress of a patient who is at risk and is receiving treatment.

Q. I had an X-ray taken recently of my shoulder and was told the bones seen on the picture were osteoporotic. Does that mean that all my bones have osteoporosis and I should expect many fractures?

A. Not necessarily. Osteoporosis may be seen in bones around a joint with arthritis or bursitis because of changes in activity of the muscles around the joint and in the circulation to the nearby bones. In such cases, the rest of the skeleton may be completely normal.

When generalized osteoporosis occurs, different bones and different parts of a bone may be affected to a different extent. A bone is composed of two types of tissue: trabecular, or net-like bone, which dissolves more easily; and cortical, or dense bone, which is more resistant. The long bones of the body, such as the humerus, femur, tibia, and radius, have relatively more cortical bone and do not show changes until much later in the process. Other bones — notably the jaw bone, the vertebrae, the heel bone, the hip bone, the ends of long bones at the wrist — have more trabecular bone and show osteoporosis early. One of the first bones to become osteoporotic is the jaw bone; demineralization here causes loosening of the teeth and a form of periodontal disease. About 40 to 50 percent of people under the age of 45 with periodontal disease go on to develop osteoporosis in the rest of the skeleton.

Q. I have cardiac angina and my doctor has prescribed "calcium channel blocker" drugs for this. I also have osteoporosis. Should I be fearful of taking high amounts of calcium?

A. No, not at all. The calcium channel blockers work at the cell walls, decreasing the concentration of calcium within the cells and producing a relaxation of smooth muscles. A low intake of calcium in the diet increases the body's production of parathyroid hormone which increases the calcium concentration in the cell, opposing the action of the drugs. A diet high in calcium may, therefore, actually make the calcium channel blocker drugs more effective.

Q. I have had lactose intolerance ever since my teens and cannot drink milk. I get violent diarrhea, stomach cramping, and just feel miserable if I drink milk or eat ice cream. I don't like taking pills and so how can I get enough calcium to prevent osteoporosis?

A. Many people, even those with severe lactose intolerance, can take small amounts — less than 4 ounces — of milk as part of a meal without more effect than softening of the stools. The fermentation processes used in the manufacture and aging of cheese also destroys lactose; one ounce of most cheeses is equivalent to an eight-ounce glass of milk in calcium content.

In addition, there are enzyme products available commerically (such as LactAid) that may be mixed with milk and after 24 hours in the refrigerator will have removed all or most of the lactose. (This makes the milk taste slightly sweet.) The enzyme substance is also available in coated tablets that can be taken with milk and milk-containing foods to help digest the lactose in the intestine. A lactose-reduced milk is available in many supermarkets as LactAid milk or Calcimilk Lactaid.

Yogurt is a form of milk in which the yogurt bacteria have digested some of the lactose. A further benefit of yogurt, if it is an "active culture" yogurt, is that the organisms continue to work in the intestine, removing even more of the lactose.

Q. In the past few years, I have been hearing a lot about osteoporosis — in newspaper and magazine articles, on television, and from my friends. Is this a new disease that has just been discovered?

A. Osteoporosis has always been around. Elderly people, particularly women, have frequently had fractures of the hips, forearms and spine due to osteoporosis. Although not everyone develops osteoporosis, it was long considered the result of normal aging until about thirty years ago, when it was found to be related to patterns of dietary intake of calcium, as well as of other nutrients influencing calcium use by the body. In recent years, as more people live to the "golden years," we have become more aware of this disorder which, while not one of the "killer diseases," produces much pain and discomfort for older people.

In addition to the increased awareness of osteoporosis on the part of both patients and health care professionals, there may also be a real increase in its incidence because of changes in Americans' patterns of eating. Since 1945, the average consumption of milk and milk products (the main sources of calcium in our diets) has dropped significantly, accompanied by increases in the use of beverages that may increase bone loss, such as colas and alcohol. Consequently, more people have been consuming diets low in calcium in the past forty years, with the result that more people in their sixties and older may be susceptible to osteoporosis.

Q. I am 40 years old and I am in excellent health. However, my mother (who is 67) recently developed back pain and was told by her doctor that her spine was deteriorating. My 71-year old aunt broke both her forearms at the wrists last year when she fell on the ice. I remember my grandmother dying from pneumonia after she broke her hip at age 69. Should I be worried about developing osteoporosis?

A. You probably *do* have a genetic tendency to develop osteoporosis. The difficulties experienced by your mother, aunt, and grandmother are frequent results of osteoporosis.

We do not know all the metabolic differences seen in the three out of ten women who do develop osteoporosis as compared with those who don't. Generally, women with reddish-blonde hair, light blue eyes, pale freckled skin that doesn't tan easily, and thin skin that bruises easily are more susceptible to bone demineralization. They frequently also have more gall-bladder disease, more emphysema, and tend to be smaller in height and weight than those who don't develop osteoporosis.

The absorption of calcium from the diet is less efficient in such individuals and they may require more vitamin D in their diets. Since vitamin D in large amounts may have life-threatening effects, extra amounts should never be taken without close medical supervision.

Q. I have high blood pressure as well as osteoporosis. Will increasing my calcium intake do anything to my blood pressure?

A. People who eat diets low in calcium tend to have higher blood pressure than those on high intakes. Increasing the intake of calcium often lowers blood pressure after several weeks to months. How this occurs is not clear. One possible explanation is that with a low dietary intake of calcium there is increased secretion of parathyroid hormone (PTH) which then raises the calcium concentration within the cells of the blood vessels and the muscles controlling their flexibility. A higher intake of calcium then lowers the PTH level which, in turn, improves the tone of the blood vessels, lowering the blood pressure.

Q. I have heard and read many conflicting opinions regarding the value of fluoride in preventing and treating osteoporosis. Does it help or is it harmful?

A. The answer is "yes it does help" and "yes it may be harmful." As with so many other drugs and nutrients, there is an amount that is beneficial, but large excesses may be toxic. When fluoride is present in the food and water as bones and teeth are formed, it is deposited in trace amounts along with calcium, making the bones and teeth stronger and more resistant to solution. This amount of flouride—1 to 2 milligrams a day—can be obtained by drinking and cooking with water that has its fluoride content adjusted to 1 ppm (1 milligram per quart).

Fluoride in much larger quantities (20 to 40 milligrams/day) has been used in the treatment of osteoporosis but there have been variable results. More bone is deposited, but only if the fluoride is accompanied by a high calcium diet and is not taken at the same time as the calcium, since it binds in the intestine with calcium, preventing both from being absorbed. If large amounts of fluoride are taken with a low calcium diet, too much fluoride is deposited in the bones making them more brittle and more easily fractured. The large doses of fluoride, furthermore, are very irritating to the stomach, particularly when taken, as they should be, without food.

Q. I have been very overweight most of my life and frequently go on semi-starvation diets to lose weight. I usually take a vitamin pill when I am dieting. Do I need extra calcium too?

A. Gaining and losing weight in a "yo-yo" pattern is bad for all of your tissues, not just your bones. When you are on a crash diet, losing weight rapidly, you also lose calcium and other essential body constituents to a greater extent than you lose body fat. Taking supplements helps prevent some vitamin and mineral losses but cannot prevent the destruction of cells and organs. When you regain the weight, you replace the fat and water you've lost, but you cannot completely rebuild the other tissues. You should try to lose weight very slowly, regularly, and keep it off, even if you cannot achieve the lowest weight you desire.

On the other hand, you are less at risk for osteoporosis than someone who is thinner than you are. Osteoporosis rarely occurs in obese people. There are several explanations for this. The higher weight is probably the result of a higher intake of food and, therefore, of calcium as well, over a long period of time, usually including adolescence and early adulthood. The higher weight imposes a greater stress on the bones, increasing their usual density. The increased body fat stores estrogen for longer periods of time, preventing the loss of bone usually seen at menopause when estrogen production drops rapidly.

Q. My mother's doctor told her she has "calcium deposits" in her shoulder. Are they caused by eating too much calcium?

A. No, calcium deposits in joints are not related to diet. When the lining of a joint is destroyed by arthritis or trauma, the body "walls off" the destroyed tissue by depositing calcium around it in the same way an oyster forms a pearl in response to irritation by a grain of sand. The calcium in these "pearls" or "joint mice" comes from the body fluids and is deposited whether or not any calcium is consumed in the diet.

Q. I am 68 years old and live in a nursing home. Sometimes I don't go out into the sun for weeks, especially during the winter. Should I be taking a supplement of vitamin D?

A. Most people's bodies make enough vitamin D for their needs just from the action of the sun's ultraviolet rays on cholesterol in the skin. In years past we saw many cases of vitamin D deficiency in people who had no exposure to sunlight. However, some types of fluorescent lights, particularly the "daylight" kind, have the same action of sunlight in forming vitamin D. If you don't get enough of either sunlight or fluorescent light you may need vitamin D supplements. The U.S. RDA is 400 International Units a day. More than that should be taken only if prescribed by a physician.

Q. I'm a vegetarian and take large doses of vitamins every day. Are these helping protect me against osteoporosis? Can too much of any one vitamin be harmful?

A. Large doses of vitamins are *never* needed by anyone. If a diet is deficient in a particular vitamin, it should be supplemented by an amount equivalent to that in a normal diet. High doses (more than 5 to 10 times the recommended daily allowances) of vitamins A and D are always harmful. High doses of vitamin C and folic acid may be harmful to some people. High doses of vitamin E over many years may also cause damage.

In osteoporosis, no vitamin alone can protect. Vitamin D is needed, but always accompanied by adequate amounts of calcium. On a diet low in calcium, even small amounts of vitamin D may actually increase bone destruction.

A completely vegetarian diet may be deficient in many substances such as calcium, iron, and vitamin B-12. A lacto-vegetarian diet is usually deficient in iron. But an ovo-lacto-vegetarian diet can be planned so that it is not deficient in anything and so no supplements of any kind would be needed.

Q. I am on prednisone for rheumatoid arthritis and my 12-year-old son takes another form of cortisone for his asthma. Will these drugs affect our calcium needs?

A. Very definitely yes. Patients with rheumatoid arthritis have an increased tendency to develop osteoporosis early in life. Prednisone and related drugs decrease the ability to absorb calcium from the intestine and also prevent normal bone formation.

Your son is at increased risk because of his age. As an adolescent, he requires more calcium for the normal growth process, as well as to compensate for the cortisone effects. Both of you should be on high calcium diets and may possibly need additional vitamin D.

Q. Whenever I take calcium supplements, I become constipated. What can I do about this?

A. Many people, particularly those over 55 years old, become constipated with new medications or changes in their diets. Others may develop diarrhea from exactly the same medications. Calcium supplements (also iron and some antacids) are frequent causes of constipation. There are several ways to avoid this problem. One is to take the supplements along with food and to maintain a diet high in fiber and liquids. This is generally good advice for all people whether or not they are taking supplements. The second approach is to take certain brands of a calcium supplement that also contains a mild laxative, such as magnesium hydroxide (Milk of Magnesia). As a rule, if the extra calcium comes from the foods that you eat, constipation does not occur.

Q. I am taking zinc supplements which I buy at the health food store. Can that help my bone health?

A. No. In fact, it may make you more likely to develop calcium deficiency and thus osteoporosis. The requirement for zinc is relatively low and an excess prevents the absorption of calcium, particularly if your diet is low in calcium. In addition, excess zinc prevents normal utilization of iron and copper in the diet. You should not take zinc supplements without consulting with your physcian.

Q. Does it make any difference when I take my calcium supplements —with meals, at bedtime, on an empty stomach?

A. Calcium is absorbed best when there is no other food in the intestines. On the other hand, since bone is made up of many other substances obtained from food, and calcium is normally obtained from the diet, it makes sense to take it with meals. In some diseases, such as osteomalacia, associated with malabsorption of calcium and vitamin D, the losses of calcium are greater at night than in the daytime. Taking extra calcium at bedtime would only increase these losses unless the underlying disease is first corrected. As a rule, because calcium is usually absorbed inefficiently at any time, exact timing of intake makes little difference.

Q. I have always eaten well-balanced meals that include milk. Now that I am 50 years old, I notice a tendency to put on weight and have cut back on the size of my portions of food. Doesn't it make sense to cut back on my calcium intake as well?

A. Although your need for calories decreases as you get older and are less active, your requirement for protein, minerals, and vitamins remains the same. For calcium in particular, the amount in the diet should actually be increased, since in both men and women there is a decrease in the efficiency of absorption by the intestine and so more has to be consumed to supply the same needs. The best way to cut back on calorie consumption is to eliminate foods low in other nutrients, such as soft drinks, desserts and fried foods, while maintaining the same intake of milk, meat, bread, fruits, and vegetables.

Q. I have osteoporosis, which has caused me to have had several fractures of my spine. My doctor has recommended that I take $1^1/_2$ grams of calcium a day because I don't drink milk or eat any milk products. Would I heal better if I doubled the dose?

A. No, you are probably taking the optimum amount already. The total amount of calcium absorbed increases as the calcium intake in the diet increases, up to about 1.2 to 1.4 grams of calcium a day. Beyond that, the body cannot absorb much more and any extra calcium you consume passes through unabsorbed. It may, in fact, lead to problems such as constipation and poor absorption of other minerals.

Q. I am 73 years old and have lost about three inches in height since I was 50. My doctor says it's because I have crushed vertebrae due to osteoporosis. If I start taking calcium and vitamin D now, will I regain any of this height?

A. Unfortunately, no. When the loss of bone has progressed to the point that bones have collapsed, osteoporosis cannot be reversed and the bones rebuilt to their previous size. If osteoporosis is detected by X-rays or bone densitometry before fractures occur, there is some chance of putting enough calcium back into the bones to avoid fractures. Osteoporosis can be prevented, unaffected bones can be preserved, and further damage to collapsed bone can be avoided by increased intake of calcium and appropriate amounts of vitamin D, but once damage has occurred, the destroyed portions cannot be repaired.

Q. I have heard that large doses of vitamin C are good for many things. Can they help prevent or treat osteoporosis?

A. In scurvy, the disease seen in severe vitamin C deficiency, changes in the bone can occur that look like osteoporosis. This occurs primarily in children. Scurvy occurs when there is failure in the normal production of the protein holding bone together. It can be prevented and treated (before fractures occur) with very small amounts of vitamin C, about 20 to 30 milligrams a day. In most people with osteoporosis, vitamin C will have no effect; certainly, large doses are not necessary. Excessively high doses, greater than 1,000 milligrams a day, may cause diarrhea and kidney stones, thus increasing the loss of calcium.

Q. I don't like taking synthetic chemicals. Wouldn't it be better to get my calcium from natural sources such as dolomite and my vitamin D from cod liver oil?

A. Dolomite is a form of limestone. Although it does contain calcium carbonate, a good source of calcium, it also contains variable amounts of other minerals that can be quite poisonous, such as arsenic, lead, cadmium, and even uranium, depending on where it was mined.

Cod liver oil is a good source of vitamin D but also contains vitamin A. If you take extra cod liver oil to increase your vitamin D intake, you may be also taking toxic amounts of vitamin A. One of the principal effects of vitamin A poisoning is destruction of bone, so you will be deteriorating rather than improving your bones. The best natural source for calcium is in foods.

Q. I am a 45-year-old woman and I work 40 to 50 hours a week running my company in addition to caring for my family. Although I eat well-balanced meals, I can only get outdoors on weekends. I'm afraid I don't get enough sunlight to make the vitamin D I need to protect me against osteoporosis. Do I need a vitamin supplement?

A. No. If you get sun exposure periodically, your skin can make enough vitamin D to last a long time. Vitamin D is not easily excreted, but is stored in the body for many weeks and months, being released as you need it.

Q. I don't drink milk, but I use non-dairy coffee whitener in my coffee and on my cereal. Do I get enough calcium that way?

A. Most non-dairy whiteners contain little or no calcium. Read the label carefully. They contain hydrogenated fats (more saturated than milk fat), sweeteners, milk protein, and various preservatives, flavoring agents, and coloring agents. Nutritionally, they are not milk replacements.

Q. I am 38 years old and have been running ten miles a day for the past five years. I enjoy running because I am competing against myself and I can feel myself unwind after a day of business problems. The only changes I've noticed are that I've lost weight, my muscles have firmed up, my periods stopped three years ago. Will the extra exercise I get from running protect me enough from osteoporosis so that I don't have to take estrogen hormone?

A. This is a controversial area. Exercise may offer additional protection against bone loss, but there is no evidence that vigorous exercise is any better for protection against osteoporosis than moderate levels of exercise such as daily walking. On the other hand, marathon runners and others who exercise excessively daily stop their menstrual periods and have low estrogen levels, which may increase bone loss. It may be that the losses of bone due to your early menopause may be partially compensated by our exercise level, but if you are forced to stop running for other reasons, you will be at increased risk. You should have your endocrine status completely evaluated for the possible need for additional hormone and you should be sure you're getting enough calcium in your diet.

Q. I am 42 years old and still have normal regular menstrual periods. My dentist told me I have severe periodontal disease with bone resorption in my jaw. Is this a form of osteoporosis and what can I do about it?

A. There are several known causes for periodontal disease and all result in infection of the gums, resorption of bone, and loss of teeth. It has been shown that in many individuals, generalized osteoporosis may show its first changes in the jaw bone with loss of the delicate supporting trabecular bone. The loss of the bone causes the teeth to loosen, producing damage to the gums and subsequent infection. The infection produces more destruction and eventual loss of the teeth.

The primary immediate treatment is to clear up the infection, as recommended by the dentist. This sometimes requires surgery. Long-term treatment of the underlying bone disease should also be started since, as mentioned above, the jaw bone changes are frequently an indication that osteoporosis is beginning in other bones, such as the spine, hips, and wrists. Dietary intake of calcium should be increased to about 1,500 milligrams a day; additional vitamin D may be necessary; fluoride intake should be checked to ensure 1 to 2 milligrams a day; and estrogen supplements should be considered when menopause occurs.

Other medical disorders cause osteoporosis and often show the signs first as periodontal disease. The principal one is diabetes, where repeated episodes of poor control cause large losses of calcium from the body. People with seizure disorders who have been taking medication for many years also develop loss of bone in the jaw and later in the spine.

PART II

WHERE TO
FIND CALCIUM

5

THE LOW CALORIE ROAD
TO HIGH CALCIUM LIVING

ALL OF US make a decision several times every day that is crucial to our health: selecting which foods to eat. Sometimes the decision is made thoughtfully, after carefully considering the alternatives. We may take five minutes or more to read the elaborate four-page menu at a gourmet restaurant. Other times we act on impulse, unable to resist the tempting aroma of the chocolate chip cookies at the shopping mall or airport.

Often circumstances beyond our control dictate what we eat. We reach for our favorite breakfast cereal and attempt to shake the contents into the bowl, only to find that the box is almost empty. So we mutter a few words about our inconsiderate teenage offspring, and stop for a danish and coffee on the way to work.

Health conscious men and women drive through sleet and snow to avoid missing their weekly exercise class, yet ponder more carefully over what to wear than what to eat. They continue to buy foods with "empty calories" —food devoid of nutrients other than calories.

Take Charge of the Calcium in Your Body!

Whatever your food patterns have been in the past, you must first assess how much calcium you are already getting before you make any drastic changes in your diet. A simple food diary kept for one week — a record of everything that you eat and drink — will provide the answer. Although you probably don't eat the same foods every day or every week, a one-week record will reveal your eating patterns (types of food and quantities).

To make your diary, take sheets of lined paper and place five headings across the top of each page: "Time Food Eaten," "Name of Food," "Amount," "Calorie Content," "Calcium Content."

Keeping the diary will be easy and will not take very much time. Keep the paper and a pencil with you, and every time you eat or drink something, fill in the first three columns. Write down every food and beverage, whether it's a snack or a "sit-down" meal. Write it down immediately. Don't wait until the end of the day to try to remember what you had for breakfast.

At the end of the day, fill in the last two columns. Use the Calcium and Calorie Counter to make your calculations. For a packaged food that is not listed, consult the nutrition information panel. Or make an estimate based on the listed contents; ingredients are listed in *decreasing order* of their weight. For example, if mozzarella cheese is listed 17th out of 20 ingredients on the package of frozen pizza, you can assume that there is very little calcium. (Later, after you have learned to "think calcium," you may want to add an ounce of grated part-skim mozzarella to your pizza, which will add 20 percent of the U.S. RDA for calcium).

The next step, after you finish filling out the information for the day, is to add up the percentages of calcium. Check the table of Recommended Daily Calcium Intake to determine whether your calcium needs are being met.

You can use the four typical food diaries that follow, and our suggested modifications, as guides for boosting your own calcium intake without increasing calories. They will show that there are many different paths to better bone health.

Four Food Diaries

When we became aware of the large gap between the dietary calcium women should have and the amount most were actually consuming, we decided to make our own survey. We contacted ten women representing different age groups and varied lifestyles, and asked each of them to keep a food diary for three days — two days during the week and one weekend day. We asked them to record every food and beverage they consumed during those days, and to include the times the foods were eaten. We did not let them know the purpose of our request, other than to say we were writing a nutrition book, because we didn't want them to increase the calcium in their diets above their normal intake level.

The completed food diaries were analyzed for nutrient content by the HVH-CWRU Nutrient Data Base at Case Western Reserve University in Cleveland, Ohio. Four one-day diaries were then selected as representative of different ages, occupations, and lifestyles.

The diaries are presented here, first, just as they were given to us. Each diary is followed by a discussion of the results of computerized nutritional analysis of that day's intake, with our specific dietary recommendations to improve the woman's calcium intake to meet the U.S. RDA of 1,000 milligrams. Each diary is then presented in a revised version with the suggested substitutions.

Guidelines used in changing the diets

1. We tried to make the food changes consistent with the individual's eating style.

2. A food that substitutes for another does not require more cooking or preparation time than the one it replaces.

3. Added or substituted foods are good sources for both calcium and other nutrients (and better than the foods they replace).

4. We used the U.S. RDA of 1,000 milligrams per day as the desirable calcium level, since it is the standard for the nutrition label information on food products.

5. We planned the daily intake to be consistent with the recommendations in "The Dietary Guidelines for Americans," issued by the U.S. Department of Agriculture and the U.S. Department of Health and Human Services, which advises Americans to:

> Eat a variety of foods.
>
> Avoid too much fat, saturated fat and cholesterol.
>
> Eat foods with adequate starch and fiber.
>
> Avoid too much sugar.
>
> Avoid too much sodium.

6. We based the calorie level on the general guidelines set by the Food and Nutrition Board's *Recommended Dietary Allowances (1980*

edition), which states that there are a "wide range of energy intakes appropriate for any group of people." The requirement for calories is extremely variable among individuals and depends on body build, activity level, energy needs, and biological stage.

The number of pounds that registers on the bathroom scale is not the only guideline for determining a desirable weight; another factor is how much fat is under the skin. A woman who is athletic and muscular may weigh more than someone with a more sedentary lifestyle who sits at a desk all day.

7. We planned the high calcium revisions of the food diaries based on the limited information that we had available: the height, weight, and occupation of each woman. Since none of them indicated any problem with high blood pressure, we made no dietary changes solely to lower sodium intake.

The women keeping the diaries were Jennifer, age 17, Sharon, age 30, Mary, age 33, and Betsy, age 47. Look over the diaries to find the one that most closely approximates your own eating patterns. Then, use the revised version to discover how easily you can substitute calcium rich foods for those with less nutritional value.

FOOD DIARY NO. 1

Name: Jennifer
Age: 17
Height: 5'5"
Weight: 125 lbs
Occupation: High school student; works weekends at an ice cream parlor.

TIME	FOOD	AMOUNT	CALORIES	CALCIUM (U.S. RDA)
7:30 AM	White toast	2 slices	138	4%
	Margarine	1 Tbsp	101	*
	Grape jelly	1 Tbsp	49	*
	2% low fat milk	1/2 cup	61	15%
11:15 AM	White bread	2 slices	138	4%
	Corned beef	2 slices	211	*
	American cheese	1 oz	107	17%
	Sauerkraut, canned	1/3 cup	14	3%
	2% chocolate milk	1 cup	179	28%
	Chocolate Zingers	3	120	4%
3:00 PM	Apple cider	1/2 cup	62	*
4:30 PM	Bacon	4 slices	178	*
4:45 PM	Ham	1 slice	79	*
	American cheese	1 oz	107	17%
	Mayonnaise	1 Tbsp	99	*
	White bread	2 slices	135	4%
	2% low fat milk	1 cup	121	30%
6:15 PM	Coca Cola	8 oz	106	*
6:45 PM	Coca Cola	8 oz	106	*
	Choc. covered peanuts	4	53	*
7:30 PM	Coca Cola	8 oz	106	*
	Choc. covered peanuts	1	13	*
	Choc. covered coconut	1	57	*
8:45 PM	Chocolate ice cream	1 scoop	148	9%
	Marshmallow toppng	1 Tbsp	137	1%
	Chocolate sprinkles	2 tsp	36	*
9:10 PM	Pistachios	11	83	2%
	Choc. covered raisins	1	4	*

Daily Intake Summary
    Total Calories: 2,748
    Total Calcium: 138% U.S. RDA

* Less than 2% U.S. RDA

Discussion of Jennifer's food diary

Jennifer's calcium intake, at 138 percent of the U.S. RDA, was just about adequate for her increased adolescent needs. The three servings of milk accounted for 78 percent of the total. Her calorie intake was 2,748, slightly higher than the 2,100 calories recommended for Jennifer's age group and height and weight.

The three 8-ounce cola drinks within an hour and a half could increase phosphorus intake to the point where it interferes with calcium absorption. Since cola drinks are "empty" calories without nutritional value, they are eliminated in her revised diet. The chocolate Zingers and some of the chocolate candy are eliminated for the same reason.

Jennifer's nutrient needs are not being met in some areas. Her vitamin C intake (at 31%) is less than a third of her daily requirement. Her vitamin A and iron are both about 25 percent below the recommended levels. The addition of half a cantaloupe at breakfast adds vitamin A, vitamin C, and iron, as well as calcium.

Although the marshmallow topping and some chocolate candy was excluded in the revised diary, the temptations of working in an ice cream store were taken into consideration.

Jennifer's revised diary (*added or replaced foods are in bold type*)

TIME	FOOD	AMOUNT	CALORIES	CALCIUM (U.S. RDA)
7:30 AM	White toast	2 slices	138	4%
	Margarine	1/2 Tbsp	50	*
	Grape jelly	1 Tbsp	49	*
	2% low fat milk	1/2 cup	61	15%
	Total whole wheat cereal	**1 oz**	**100**	**20%**
	Cantaloupe	**1/2**	**95**	**3%**
11:15 AM	White bread	2 slices	138	4%
	Corned beef	2 slices	211	*
	American cheese	1 oz	107	17%
	Sauerkraut	1/3 cup	14	3%
	2% chocolate milk	1 cup	179	28%
3:00 PM	Apple cider	1/2 cup	62	*
4:30 PM	Bacon	4 slices	178	*
4:45 PM	Ham	1 slice	79	*
	American cheese	1 oz	107	17%
	Mayonnaise	1 Tbsp	99	*
	Whole wheat bread	**2 slices**	**130**	**4%**
	2% low fat milk	1 cup	121	30%
6:45 PM	**2% low fat milk**	**6 oz**	**114**	**23%**
	Chocolate syrup	**1 Tbsp**	**46**	*
	Soda water	**2 oz**	**0**	*
7:30 PM	Choc. covered peanuts	4	53	*
8:45 PM	Chocolate ice cream	1 scoop	148	9%
	Chocolate sprinkles	2 tsp	36	*
9:10 PM	Pistachios	11	83	2%
	Choc. covered raisin	1	4	*

Daily Intake Summary:
    Total calories: 2,402
    Total calcium: 179% U.S. RDA
    Revised diary has 346 fewer calories and 41% more calcium.

* Less than 2% U.S. RDA

FOOD DIARY NO. 2

Name: Mary
Age: 33
Height: 4'11"
Weight: 95 lbs
Occupation: Houseparent at group home for retarded children.

TIME	FOOD	AMOUNT	CALORIES	CALCIUM (U.S. RDA)
9:30 AM	Wheat bread	1 slice	65	2%
10:15 PM	Candy	1/4 oz	26	*
12:45 PM	Fish sandwich (Burger King)	1	488	5%
	Onion rings	1 portion	274	12%
1:40 PM	Herbal tea	1 cup	0	*
5:30 PM	Spaghetti w/meat sauce	2 cups	660	25%
	Green beans	2/3 cup	20	4%
8:40 PM	Herbal tea	1 cup	0	*
12:15 AM	Pepsi-Free	8 oz	0	*
	Candy	1/4 oz	26	*

Daily Intake Summary
    Total calories: 1,559
    Total calcium: 48% U.S. RDA

* Less than 2% U.S. RDA

Discussion of Mary's food diary

Mary's small size ranks her in the lower range of calorie requirements for her age group. She needs about 1,600 - 1,700 calories, which is just about what she recorded. Her calcium intake, however, at 48% of the U.S. RDA was far lower than it should be. She also fell below recommendations for iron, vitamin A, and vitamin C.

In the revised diary, we added calcium with cereal and milk, cheese to her fish sandwich, and we replaced the onion rings with a vanilla shake, which contains 30% of the U.S. RDA for calcium. The cantaloupe provides vitamins A and C as well as iron. Finally, by adding a spoonful of Parmesan cheese to the spaghetti and topping the cantaloupe with flavored yogurt, we were able to reach her recommended level of calcium.

Mary's revised food diary *(added or replaced foods are in bold type)*

TIME	FOOD	AMOUNT	CALORIES	CALCIUM (U.S. RDA)
9:30 AM	Wheat bread	1 slice	65	2%
	Total whole wheat cereal	**1 oz**	**110**	**20%**
	2% low fat milk	**¹/₂ cup**	**60**	**15%**
10:15 PM	Candy	¹/₄ oz	26	*
12:45 PM	Fish sandwich w/cheese (Burger King)	1	530	12%
	Vanilla shake	**1**	**321**	**30%**
1:40 PM	Herbal tea	1 cup	0	*
5:30 PM	Spaghetti w/meat sauce	1 cup	330	12%
	Parmesan cheese, grated	**1 Tbsp**	**25**	**7%**
	Green beans	²/₃ cup	20	4%
8:40 PM	**Cantaloupe**	**1/2**	**95**	**3%**
	Lemon or vanilla yogurt	**¹/₂ cup**	**100**	**17%**
12:15 AM	Herbal tea	8 oz	0	*

Daily Intake Summary
    Total calories: 1,682
    Total calcium: 122% U.S. RDA
    The revised diary has 123 more calories and 74% more calcium.

* Less than 2% U.S. RDA

FOOD DIARY NO. 3

Name: Sharon
Age: 30
Height: 5'3"
Weight: 115 lbs
Occupation: Administrative assistant at a mental health center; also attends graduate school.

TIME	FOOD	AMOUNT	CALORIES	CALCIUM (U.S. RDA)
7:30 AM	Apple cider	8 oz	124	*
	Cocoa (made w/water)	8 oz	110	11%
	Chocolate chip cookies	4	138	*
1:00 PM	Hot dogs (beef)	2	365	*
	Baked beans	6 oz	255	10%
	Cheese puffs	2 1/2 oz	391	4%
	Apple	1	81	*
4:30 PM	Coffee	2 cups	2	*
	Coffee whitener	2 tsp	20	*
	Sugar	1 tsp	15	*
	Apple	1	81	*
5:30 PM	Cheese puffs	1 1/2 oz	234	2%
	Chocolate crunch bar	1	136	2%
	Pepsi Cola	10 oz	132	*
8:30 PM	Lima beans	6 oz	168	3%
	Butter	1 Tbsp	101	*
	Apple cider	8 oz	124	*

Daily Intake Summary
   Total calories: 2,477
   Total calcium: 32% U.S. RDA

* Less than 2% U.S. RDA

Discussion of Sharon's food diary

Sharon has a sedentary life style, which makes her calorie intake of 2,477 too high for her height and weight. Moreover, about 40 percent of these calories are in high-calorie foods that supply few nutrients. The cheese puffs, which she nibbled while working at her desk, accounted for 625 calories — about one-fourth of the total. These are eliminated in the revised diary, along with the cookies, candy bar, and cola drink.

Sharon's calcium intake was only 32 percent of the U.S. RDA. We tried to remedy that without making drastic changes in her diet. We suggested breakfast yogurt, and preparing cocoa with milk instead of water. The candy bar is replaced with chocolate pudding, to satisfy her craving for chocolate with 10 percent more calcium, and the ice cream dessert at dinner contains 10 percent more calcium than the cookies Sharon ate for breakfast.

Sharon's intake of vitamin A was below recommended levels, so we replaced lima beans with broccoli, which is rich in calcium and vitamin A, and added vitamin A-rich carrot sticks.

Since Sharon works full time and attends graduate school, she has little time or energy to expend on food preparation. Therefore, the foods chosen as substitutions are either frozen or canned.

Sharon's revised food diary *(added or replaced foods are in bold type)*

TIME	FOOD	AMOUNT	CALORIES	CALCIUM (U.S. RDA)
7:30 AM	Apple cider	8 oz	124	*
	Cocoa (made w/skim milk)	**8 oz**	**123**	**30%**
	Breakfast yogurt			
	(Yoplait apple cinnamon)	**6 oz**	**220**	**50%**
1:00 PM	Hot dogs (beef)	2	365	*
	Cheddar cheese			
	(melted on hot dog)	**1 slice**	**110**	**20%**
	Baked beans	6 oz	255	10%
	Carrot sticks	**6**	**12**	*
	Apple	1	81	*
4:30 PM	Coffee	2 cups	2	*
	Nonfat dry milk	**2 tsp**	**10**	**3%**
	Sugar	1 tsp	15	*
	Apple	1	81	*
5:30 PM	**Chocolate pudding (can)**	**5 oz**	**160**	**10%**
8:30 PM	Apple cider	8 oz	124	*
	Pizza (Celeste 19 oz.			
	Canadian style bacon)	**¼ pizza**	**288**	**30%**
	Broccoli cuts (BirdsEye)	**3.3 oz**	**25**	**6%**
	Chocolate chip ice cream	**½ cup**	**170**	**10%**

Daily Intake Summary
    Total calories: 2,165
    Total calcium: 169% U.S. RDA
    The revised diary has 312 fewer calories and 137% more calcium.

* Less than 2% U.S. RDA

FOOD DIARY NO. 4

Name: Betsy
Age: 47
Height: 5'5"
Weight: 118 lbs
Occupation: Development director for community health agency. While keeping the food diary she was in training for the New York City Marathon.

TIME	FOOD	AMOUNT	CALORIES	CALCIUM (U.S. RDA)
9:15 AM	Banana	1	70	*
	Instant oatmeal w/raisins	1 pkg	160	10%
	Skim milk	$\frac{1}{4}$ cup	21	7%
	Coffee	$1\frac{1}{2}$ cups	4	*
10:30 AM	Diet cola	12 oz	0	*
12:00 noon	Mozzarella cheese	1 oz	80	15%
	Wheat bread	2 slices	112	4%
	Diet cola	12 oz	0	*
1:30 PM	Hershey Kisses	6	150	6%
4:30 PM	Tootsie Rolls	3	89	*
6:00 PM	Triscuit crackers	2	38	*
7:00 PM	Flank steak	1 slice	159	*
	Baked potato	$1\frac{1}{2}$	217	*
	Margarine	2 Tbsp	198	*
	Romaine lettuce	2 cups	20	7%
	Oil	2 Tbsp	240	*
	Vinegar	$\frac{1}{2}$ Tbsp	0	*
	Parmesan cheese	1 Tbsp	23	7%
8:50 PM	Hershey Kisses	4	100	4%

Daily Intake Summary
   Total calories: 1,681
   Total calcium: 60% U.S. RDA

* Less than 2% U.S. RDA

73

Discussion of Betsy's food diary

Betsy's calorie intake was insufficient to meet her unusually high energy needs while training for the marathon, and she was losing weight. During the training period she should have been getting about 2,400 calories. The revised diary increases her calories to about 2,000, the approximate amount she requires when she is not in training, but running regularly three times a week.

Betsy's calcium intake was only 60 percent of the U.S. RDA. It was increased with the addition of oyster stew (prepared with milk), Swiss cheese on the crackers, and yogurt on the baked potato.

To replace some of the chocolate candy and increase the calcium further, we added chocolate pudding. Substituting dried figs for a "candy break" also gives Betsy added calcium. Although Betsy's vitamin D intake was only 53 percent of the recommended amount, she gets enough vitamin D since she is outdoors so much.

Betsy's revised food diary (added or replaced foods are in bold type)

TIME	FOOD	AMOUNT	CALORIES	CALCIUM (U.S. RDA)
9:15 AM	Banana	1	70	*
	Instant oatmeal w/raisins	1 pkg	160	10%
	Skim milk	1/2 cup	43	15%
	Coffee	1 1/2 cups	4	*
10:30 AM	Diet cola	12 oz	0	*
12:00 noon	**Oyster stew (Campbells) 8 oz can, made w/milk**		**150**	**10%**
	Wheat bread	2 slices	112	4%
	Orange juice	**6 oz**	**90**	**2%**
1:30 PM	Hershey kisses	6	150	6%
4:30 PM	**Calimyrna figs**	**3**	**144**	**8%**
6:00 PM	Triscuit crackers	2	38	*
	Swiss cheese	**1 oz**	**110**	**20%**
7:00 PM	Flank steak	1 slice	159	*
	Baked potato	1 1/2	217	*
	Plain yogurt	**1/2 cup**	**75**	**20%**
	Romaine lettuce	2 cups	20	7%
	Oil	2 Tbsp	240	*
	Vinegar	1/2 Tbsp	0	*
	Parmesan cheese, grated	1 Tbsp	23	7%
8:50 PM	**Chocolate pudding**	**1/2 cup**	**180**	**15%**
	Skim milk	**1/2 cup**	**43**	**15%**

Daily Intake Summary
    Total calories: 2,028
    Total calcium: 139% U.S. RDA
    The revised diary has 347 more calories and 79% more calcium.

* Less than 2% U.S. RDA

6

A CALCIUM HIGH
AT THE SUPERMARKET

EVERY TIME you wheel your shopping cart through the supermarket, you have a new opportunity to start getting a higher calcium yield from your food dollars. Use the Calcium and Calorie Counter (Chapter 11) to plan ahead as you make out your shopping list.

The information that follows is given by supermarket department: dairy, frozen foods, grocery, and produce (which includes information about tofu), and pharmacy, a discussion of calcium supplement pills.

Dairy Department

The dairy case is the best place to start because it offers a multitude of calcium treasures to build bones. Milk and milk products are our best nutritional sources of calcium, not only because of the significant amount of the mineral present, but also because of the calcium to phosphorus ratio, which is conducive to skeletal growth, and the presence of nutrients such as vitamin D (if fortified) and lactose, which favor calcium absorption.

Cheese

There are Federal regulations that set standards for the production of cheese. A cheese may be labeled *natural* if it is made from a dairy product, with enzymes, and undergoes a natural aging process. *Processed cheese* and *cheese foods* are made from cheeses.

A *cheese substitute* must be "nutritionally equal" to the natural cheese it replaces in every nutrient but fat and calories, and it must have a

77

nutrition information label and a statement of ingredients. It may contain excessive amounts of sugar for anyone with diabetes.

An *imitation cheese* will probably be "nutritionally inferior" (meaning it does not contain the major nutrients contained in natural cheese). Imitation cheese need not have a nutrition information label. If you're trying to boost your calcium intake, a natural, processed, or substitute cheese is a better choice than an imitation cheese.

A single ounce of cheese can bring you 20 to 30 percent closer to your daily calcium goal. With so many varieties available, cheese is one of the best choices to boost your daily calcium intake. Natural Swiss should head your shopping list — a 1-ounce serving may provide 30 percent of the U.S. RDA for calcium and 110 calories. Other popular cheeses are Cheddar and Monterey Jack (20% calcium, 110 calories) and part-skim mozzarella (20% calcium, 80 calories).

Processed Swiss cheese contains slightly less calcium (20%) than natural Swiss and fewer calories (90); however, the higher sodium content (420 mg in one ounce compared to 75 mg in natural Swiss) may interfere with calcium absorption. Similarly, pasturized process American cheese contains slightly less calcium and more sodium than the Cheddar cheese from which it is made, as does pasturized process American cheese food and spread.

Lowfat cottage cheese is a frequent lunch choice for many waistline-watchers, who assume that because it is a dairy product it must be a rich source of calcium. The fact is that the calcium content of cottage cheese varies considerably, and a 4-ounce serving may range from 4 percent to 15 percent of the U.S. RDA. When buying cottage cheese or ricotta cheese, check for the calcium content on the nutrition information label. Ricotta is richer in calcium than cottage cheese, and higher in calories. Part-skim ricotta is preferred by calorie watchers.

Milk

Milk is one of the best sources of calcium, providing 30 percent of the U.S. RDA in each 8-ounce serving. The added "bones bonus" in milk is the combination of lactose and vitamin D (contained in fortified milk), which improves the body's ability to absorb calcium. Milk also has an almost ideal balance of phosphorus to calcium and contains healthful vitamins.

Choose the type of milk with the calorie and milkfat content that best meets your energy needs. Drink it, pour it over cereal, and use it to make cream sauces, cream soups, custards, and puddings. Try buttermilk in soups and salad dressings. One cup of buttermilk has just 100 calories, the same as 1 percent low fat milk.

Yogurt

One of the most popular weapons against osteoporosis is yogurt. Yogurt offers a high concentration of calcium, with a serving of some brands supplying 40 to 50 percent of the U.S. RDA for calcium. Now available in an almost limitless variety of textures and flavors, yogurt makes a nutritious and palatable snack for all ages, from toddlers to seniors. It is a versatile ingredient in cooling summer soups, breakfast shakes, and many main course entrees.

Some individuals who are lactose intolerant may experience fewer digestive difficulties with yogurt, especially when they choose a brand that is labeled "with active yogurt cultures." Heating, however, destroys the beneficial bacteria in the active cultures.

You can easily make a nonfat or low fat, low calorie yogurt product in your own kitchen: *yogurt cream cheese*, a look-alike and taste-alike for commercial cream cheese. Instructions for making yogurt cream cheese are in Chapter 8.

Frozen Foods

Don't forget to stop by the frozen foods cases, because many frozen products are high in calcium content. Among entrees and dinners are such favorites as macaroni and cheese, pizza, lasagna, veal parmesan, and cheese enchiladas.

The calcium-rich frozen vegetables include broccoli, kale, collards, mustard greens, okra, and spinach. Some varieties will be higher in calcium, and some lower, than their fresh counterparts. Vegetables in cream or cheese sauces will have added calcium; those in butter sauces will only have more calories.

The calcium in ice cream, frozen yogurt, and other frozen desserts is variable; it may range from 4 to 20 percent. A half-cup serving of vanilla ice cream, for example, may contain from 8 to 20 percent of the the U.S. RDA for calcium.

Grocery Department

Beans

Put a few cans of baked beans in your shopping cart before you leave the supermarket. Depending on the brand you choose, a 1-cup serving will supply between 4 and 15 percent of the U.S. RDA for calcium. Dry beans are another good source. Stock up on several packages to use in soups and casseroles and Mexican dishes. A cup of Great Northern or navy beans provides about 10 percent of the U.S. RDA for calcium.

Breads and cereals

The calcium in breads and cereals is influenced not only by the kind of flour used, but also by the addition of enrichment ingredients such as nonfat dry milk and calcium salts. Dry and hot cereals may range from less than 2 percent, to 20 percent for a "calcium-enriched" cereal. The half-cup of milk poured over the cereal adds 15 percent of the U.S. RDA. Several brands of flour are now calcium-enriched, with one cup containing 20 percent of the U.S. RDA for calcium.

Fish

Canned *salmon* is usually prominently listed among the foods that are good sources of calcium. Keep in mind the important fact that *the calcium is in the bones*, so don't pick the bones out of the salmon before serving; $3^1/2$ ounces of canned salmon contain between 15 and 20 percent of the U.S. RDA, depending on the variety. Add a can to your favorite noodle or macaroni casserole for a tasty calcium booster. (Unlike its canned counterpart, *fresh salmon* is not a good source for calcium because the bones are not softened and edible, as they are in canned salmon.)

Read the labels on the *sardine* cans, and select only the ones that are *not* skinless and boneless. One small tin (usually $3^3/4$ ounces) supplies about 30 percent of the U.S. RDA for calcium. A $7^1/2$ ounce can of Del Monte sardines in tomato sauce contains 100 percent of the U.S. RDA for calciulm. That's a lot of calcium in a little fish. Remember, again, that the calcium is in the bones.

Canned *shrimp* contains 10 percent calcium and 100 calories in a 3-ounce serving, according to USDA information.

Fruits, dried

Dried figs can hardly be classified as a low calorie food, though they are a good source of calcium. They do satisfy a craving for sweets, however, and are more nutritious than candy for between-meal snacks. Since they often have a laxative effect, they may be beneficial for adults with constipation problems, but children should eat only modest amounts.

Milk

Canned evaporated milk is a convenient food to keep on your pantry shelf. It is available in a wide variety of calorie choices: regular, low fat, and nonfat skim. Canned evaporated skimmed milk makes a creamy base for soups, cream sauces, and custards and, when refrigerated, may be whipped like whipping cream, at a fraction of the calories and cost.

Nonfat dry milk is an economical and palatable form of milk that, when mixed with other ingredients, cannot be detected by even the most avid milk-hater in the family. Each tablespoon contains 52 milligrams of calcium and only 15 calories. It can be added to fluid milk and yogurt to increase the calcium, in addition to cream sauces, mashed and scalloped potatoes, scrambled eggs, puddings, and hot cocoa, and it can be mixed into broths to convert them to cream soups. It can also be whipped for a low calorie, nonfat dessert topping. (See recipes in chapter 10.)

Those who are lactose intolerant should be aware that the concentrated lactose in nonfat dry milk or canned evaporated milk may affect them adversely.

Nuts and seeds

Although some varieties of nuts and seeds are good sources of calcium, it takes a large quanty to make much of a dent in daily calcium requirements. For example, you would have to eat about one-fourth cup of slivered almonds to fulfill 9 percent of the U.S. RDA for calcium. Nuts are also high in calories (those almonds contain 199 calories). Some physicians recommend that older patients avoid eating nuts and seeds to avoid any possibility of diverticulosis.

Puddings

A package of pudding mix, prepared as directed, contains one-half cup of milk, which adds 15 percent of the U.S. RDA to your daily calcium. Canned puddings vary in calcium from 4 to 10 percent, depending on the brand and flavor.

Soup

When your grandmother served a steaming hot bowl of cream of mushroom soup and urged you to eat it because "it's good for you," she was right. The milk in the soup was a good source of calcium. Canned "cream" soups are different from your grandmother's; most of them are poor sources of calcium unless you add milk instead of water to the contents of the can. The calcium in one 8-ounce serving will be raised to at least 15 percent of the U.S. RDA with the addition of four ounces of any kind of milk.

Processed soups, of any variety, are very high in sodium. Instead of relying on canned or dry packaged soups, make your own!

Produce Department

The produce department is where you'll find some of the best sources of calcium. The following vegetables are the highest in calcium content.

VEGETABLE (1 CUP)	CALCIUM (% U.S. RDA)	CALORIES
Beet greens, 1" pieces	16%	40
Broccoli, chopped	18%	46
Chard, Swiss, chopped	10%	36
Chinese cabbage (bok choy) shredded	16%	20
Collards, chopped	15%	26
Kale, chopped	9%	41
Kale, Scotch, chopped	17%	37
Mustard greens, chopped	10%	21
Spinach	24%	41
Okra, slices	10%	50
Turnip greens, chopped	20%	29

Sometimes it's difficult to know how much to purchase when buying vegetables. The pound of curly spinach leaves in the plastic bag looks like a huge amount, certainly more than enough to serve four people. But when you cook it for dinner, the spinach "wilts" to such a small volume it barely serves two.

The table below will help you determine the amount of raw vegetables that you need to buy to have four half-cup servings of cooked vegetable.

VEGETABLE	SUGGESTED QUANTITY
Beet greens	2 pounds
Broccoli	$1^1/_2$ pounds
Bok choy	1 pound
Collards	$1^1/_2$ pounds
Kale	$1^1/_2$ pounds
Mustard greens	$1^1/_4$ pounds
Okra	1 pound
Spinach	$1^1/_2$ pounds
Swiss chard	1 pound
Turnip greens	2 pounds

Bok Choy

This vegetable is also known as pak choy or Chinese cabbage. It bears some resemblance to a thick bunch of celery, but the stalks are smooth, not ribbed, and the leaves are darker green. Its taste and texture make it a versatile ingredient for many dishes. Bok choy is high in essential nutrients and provides, in a 1-cup cooked serving, 16 percent of the U.S. RDA for calcium, 42 percent for vitamin A, and 48 percent for vitamin C. All this is only 20 calories!

Broccoli

Broccoli is one of the best calcium bargains, with one spear (cooked, from raw) containing 21 percent of the U.S. RDA for calcium. The leaves should be cooked along with the flowerets and stems.

Fresh broccoli has more calcium per serving than most brands of plain frozen broccoli. It also provides a nutritional vitamin bonus: just one spear contains 51 percent of the U.S. RDA for vitamin A and almost twice the daily requirement (188%) for vitamin C. Broccoli is a good source of both fiber and beta-carotene, which may help guard against cancer.

Greens

"Greens" is a word used in the South to refer to collards, kale, beet greens, mustard greens, turnip greens, and Swiss chard. These vegetables are usually tied in bunches and piled high on the produce counter.

If you are not familiar with greens, ask someone in the produce department to help you identify the different types. Soon you'll be able to distinguish between the flat-leaved collard greens and the tightly-curled kale leaves, which, in turn, are different from the ruffled leaves of the mustard greens. Try one variety at a time to start; later you may want to cook several together. After you've determined which types your family likes best, you can use them to replace other vegetables in your recipes.

Greens are full of calcium and other valuable vitamins and minerals. Collards, for example, provide in a 1-cup cooked serving, 15 percent of the U.S. RDA for calcium, 84 percent for vitamin A, and only 27 calories. All the greens give you so many nutrients for your food dollar, you'll probably help yourself to several bunches.

Okra

Fried okra, dipped in cornmeal, is a traditional Southern favorite. Okra is the essential ingredient to thicken a gumbo. Eight okra pods contain 5 percent of the U.S. RDA for calcium, at only 27 calories.

Rhubarb

A cooked half-cup serving of rhubarb provides 11 percent of the U.S. RDA for calcium and, if no sugar is added, only 13 calories. Rhubarb contains oxalic acid, but the amount is reduced by cooking with added lemon juice.

Spinach

Spinach is one of the best non-dairy sources for calcium, with one cup, cooked, providing 24 percent of the U.S. RDA. A 1-cup serving also contains a wealth of other valuable nutrients: almost 300 percent of the U.S. RDA for vitamin A, 36 percent for iron, and 30 percent for vitamin C. Spinach is a better source of calcium when it is eaten cooked, rather than raw, since the amount of oxalic acid is reduced by cooking, especially when lemon juice or vinegar is added to the cooking water.

Tofu

Tofu tastes best when freshest, so buy it just before you plan to use it. Check the date on the carton, which is usually about three weeks after manufacture. Whether the tofu is in a plastic tub or a vacuum-sealed package, it is a perishable product and should always be refrigerated. Although many people believe that all tofu is high in calcium, that isn't always the case.

TOFU IS TERRIFIC, BUT . . .

Many nutritionists and health writers have recommended tofu as a good source of calcium because they received their data from a U.S. Department of Agriculture publication that lists tofu as having 85 calories and 108 milligrams of calcium (10 percent of the U.S. RDA) in a piece measuring $2^{1}/_{2}$ x $2^{3}/_{4}$ x 1 inch.

Unfortunately, there are no footnotes to explain a most important fact: *the calcium varies from one brand of tofu to another*. Although two cakes of tofu (each from a different manufacturer) may appear to be identical, a 4-ounce serving of one brand might fulfill 30 percent of your daily needs; the other only 4 percent. The variability among brands may be somewhat disconcerting to Americans, who are used to foods regulated by federal standards, with similar nutritional contents throughout the country. There are no federal regulations governing the manufacture of tofu, however.

What Makes One Tofu Different from Another? The process of making tofu is similar to that used in making cheese. Dairy farmers add a coagulant to cow's milk (or goat's milk) to separate it into curds (solid cheese) and whey (the drained liquid). Tofu is made with soymilk extracted from soybeans, and the tofu maker uses a coagulant to separate the soymilk into curds (tofu) and whey (the drained liquid). The coagulant is usually one of two types:

1. *Nigari*, which is sometimes referred to as "bittern," is extracted

from sea water. Its main active ingredient is magnesium chloride. Tofu that uses nigari as the only coagulant contains only a small amount of calcium.

2. The second is a calcium "salt," which is either *calcium sulfate*, also known as "gypsum," or *calcium chloride*. Either of these increases the calcium content significantly —more than three and a half times, according to the Standards Committee of the Soyfoods Association.

Fortunately, many tofu makers are responding to the current public concern about osteoporosis by adding calcium sulfate to their nigari-type tofu, or by switching completely to calcium sulfate as the coagulant.

William Shurtleff and Akiko Aoyagi, authors of the authoritative guide, *The Book of Tofu*, no longer recommend tofu made with nigari, as they once did. "We strongly support the use of tofu curded with calcium sulfate," Shurtleff asserts, "because of its low cost, high content of essential natural calcium, and good flavor." They are concerned that strict vegetarians who do not consume dairy products may increase their chances of getting osteoporosis if their major protein source is a tofu that is not made with calcium sulfate or calcium chloride.

A testimonial for choosing tofu made with calcium sulfate or calcium chloride comes from "Bob," a 43-year-old vegetarian who had for years relied on tofu as a major protein source:

> While I was ice-skating with my niece, I took a gentle fall and felt excruciating pain in my upper right leg. I went to the local hospital, where an X-ray revealed that I had broken the neck of my right femur, the massive thigh bone, about three inches below its top. Since this bone cannot be easily set by use of a cast, the doctor, a highly recommended orthopedic surgeon, operated and set the bone with the standard stainless steel plate and screws.
>
> On one of his visits to me in the hospital, he told me two important things. The first was that a man of my age should find it virtually impossible to break this bone, except perhaps in a serious car accident. Second, he said that as he was drilling the bone to set the screws, he noticed that the bone was exceptionally soft; he compared it with "drilling into balsa wood." He urged me to see an endocrinologist to find the cause of my brittle, soft bone.
>
> The endocrinologist, who had a strong background in nutrition, interviewed me about my diet and lifestyle, gave me a physical exam, did urine and blood analyses, and did a bone mineral density reading (with a densitometer). The densitometer results showed that my bones were

of very low density; in other words, they were quite porous. He said that for men my age, only one in a hundred had a lower bone density than I did.

According to the endocrinologist, all of the tests showed that my diet and health were otherwise good, but that for many years I had had a serious calcium imbalance caused by insufficient dietary calcium. Thus my body was forced to draw reserves out of my bones, which demineralized them until they became so weak that they broke from a minor ice skating fall.

An examination of my diet revealed that I had consumed very little dairy products over the years, and my calcium intake had been far below the RDA of 800 milligrams. I had paid careful attention to protein intake, but very little to calcium.

The endocrinologist said I should start immediately to substantially increase calcium in order to remineralize and strengthen my weak bones. Otherwise, another minor fall could easily cause another fracture. He recommended 800 milligrams of calcium a day from my diet, and adding oyster-shell calcium with vitamin D at breakfast and lunch. I am complying by drinking two glasses of low fat milk a day and consuming more sesame seeds, kale, broccoli and tofu coagulated with calcium sulfate, plus some sea vegetables.

For me, learning that I developed osteoporosis — almost certainly because of a dietary deficiency in calcium — has been a most humbling and surprising experience. I had always thought that if I ate a traditional diet I would be in the best of health. Live and learn.

How Can You Protect Yourself? Before buying tofu, be sure to read the label carefully. If there is a nutrition information label, this means that the manufacturer has voluntarily had the contents analyzed by an independent laboratory. If there is none, check the ingredients. A tofu that lists *nigari* as the only coagulant is a poor source of calcium. If you select a brand that uses *calcium sulfate* or *calcium chloride* as the coagulant, a serving may range between 15 and 30 percent of the U.S. RDA for calcium. When both types of coagulant are listed, you have no way of knowing the amount of either, so you can't know the calcium content, and you therefore cannot rely on that tofu as a good calcium source.

Don't make the mistake of thinking that all products with tofu are rich in calcium. The sweet custardy swirls of Tofutti and other frozen desserts with tofu contain hardly any calcium, through they can be a treat for those who are lactose intolerant and cannot eat ice cream.

Pharmacy: Calcium Supplement Pills

Even though you follow a high-calcium dietary life style, you may want to supplement your diet with pills on those days that your calcium intake falls below its usual level.

Calcium supplement pills should not be taken without consulting your physician, even though they are available at any drug store without a prescription. Some individuals have a tendency to form kidney stones; this may be accelerated and lead to permanent kidney damage if intake of calcium is increased. *If you or a blood relative has had a kidney stone in the past, you should not increase your intake of calcium, whether in pills or in food, without the approval of your physician.*

The calcium compounds used in supplement pills contain varying amounts of calcium. The calcium in each pill is *only a percentage* of the calcium compound the pill contains. Use the following table as a general guideline to assess the actual calcium in supplement products.

FORM OF CALCIUM	% OF CALCIUM	HOW ABSORBED?
Calcium carbonate	40%	Readily absorbed
Calcium citrate	27%	Readily absorbed
Calcium gluconate	9%	Readily absorbed
Calcium lactate	13%	Readily absorbed
Calcium phosphate	29%	Poorly absorbed

You will need to consider these percentages when reading the label of any calcium supplement product. Many women, for example take two Tums a day in the belief that they are consuming 1,000 mg of calcium, since the Tums label reads, "Active ingredient: calcium carbonate, 500 mg." Each tablet, however, contains only 200 mg of calcium (40% of 500 mg). So it is necessary to take five Tums to consume 1,000 mg of calcium.

Calcium carbonate is the most concentrated form of calcium and the one most readily absorbable, although in high doses it may cause constipation or flatulence. Calcium gluconate is less constipating, but many more pills must be taken for the same amount of calcium.

Calcium supplements that are advertised as "natural limestone" should be avoided because they may be contaminated with lead and other toxic elements. Two other types of calcium supplements, usually sold in health food stores, are bone-meal and dolomite. These contain other minerals, in addition to the calcium, which may be toxic.

The actual availability of the calcium in a specific brand of a supplement may also depend on the effect of the manufacturing process on the disintegration of the table and its dissolution in the body. A recent study by Drs. C. J. Carr and R. F. Shangraw of the University of Maryland has shown that different brands of calcium carbonate, when stirred in solutions of acid similar to that in the stomach, may not release the same amount of calcium. For instance, Os-Cal (oyster shell), Suplical (chewable calcium carbonate), and Tums (calcium carbonate) release about 100 percent of the calcium in one hour. Other brands, while showing the same ingredients on the labels, released only 5 to 70 percent under the same conditions. Some of these results are shown below.

NAME OF PRODUCT	DISTRIBUTOR	DISSOLVED IN 30 MIN
Os-Cal 500	Marion Labs, Inc.	88%
Suplical	Warner-Lambert	98%
Tums	Norcliff-Thayer	100%
Caltrate-600	Lederle Labs	69%
Oyster Shell Calcium w/vit. D	AARP Pharmacy Serv.	8%
Potent Calcium 600 mg	General Nutrition	5%
Nature's GLO High Potency Calcium Formula	L. Perrigo Co.	67%
Biocal	Miles Labs, Inc.	5%
Calcium as Carbonate	Rite Aid Corp.	7%

Some pharmaceutical manufacturers include vitamin D in their supplements, since vitamin D (in its active form) stimulates intestinal absorption of calcium. However, the number of pills needed to fulfill your daily calcium requirement may contain far more than 400 IU, which is the U.S. RDA for vitamin D. Too much vitamin D (more than 1,000 IU per day) may have harmful effects, including bone loss. So consult your doctor to determine your individual needs for vitamin D as well as for calcium.

The following table can help you, in consulting with your physician, to make choices about calcium supplements.

NAME OF PRODUCT	FORM OF CALCIUM	MG CALCIUM PER TABLET	NO. TABLETS FOR 1,000 MG	VIT. D. PER TABLET
Avail	Carbonate	400	2 1/2	400 IU
Biocal	Carbonate	250	4	---
Biocal	Carbonate	500	2	---
Caladay	Carbonate	667	1 1/2	---
Calcet	Gluconate, carbonate, lactate	152.8	6 1/2	---
Calcet Plus	Carbonate	152.8	6 1/2	400 IU
Calicaps	Carbonate, gluconate, phosphate	125	8	67 IU
Cal-El-D	Carbonate	500	2	200 IU
Cal-Sup 600	Carbonate	600	1 1/2+	200 IU
Cal-Sup 600 Plus	Carbonate	600	1 1/2+	200 IU
Caltrate 600	Carbonate	600	1 1/2+	---
Caltrate 600 + Iron/Vit. D	Carbonate	600	1 1/2+	125 IU
Caltrate 600 + D	Carbonate	600	1 1/2+	125 IU
Citracal	Citrate	200	5	---
Di-Cal D w/Vit C	Phosphate	117	8+	133 IU
Di-Cal D Wafers	Phosphate	232	4+	200 IU
Os-Cal 500	Carbonate	500	2	---
Os-Cal 250	Carbonate	250	4	125 IU
Osteo-Cal	Carbonate	600	1 1/2+	125 IU
Posture	Phosphate	600	1 1/2+	
Posture-D	Phosphate	600	1 1/2+	250 IU
Suplical	Carbonate	600	1 1/2+	---
Theracal	Carbonate	334	3	---

Antacids

Some antacids, like those listed below, may be recommended by your doctor as a calcium supplement. However, some types of antacids may interfere with the absorption of calcium because they contain aluminum. Popular brands that contain aluminum are Di-Gel, Gaviscon, Gelusil, Maalox, Mylanta, Rolaids, and Tempo.

The following antacids *do not* contain aluminum.

WHERE TO FIND CALCIUM

ANTACID	CALCIUM	TABLETS PER DAY FOR FOR 1,000 MG CALCIUM
Alka Mints	340 mg	3
Calcitrel	234 mg	4+
Chooz	200 mg	5
Titralac	168 mg	6
Tums	200 mg	5
Tums E-X	300 mg	3+

7
GROWING CALCIUM IN YOUR GARDEN

THE VEGETABLES that are the highest in calcium are among the easiest to grow, even for the beginning gardener. All you need are a few feet in your backyard that you can dig up to make a garden. You will be amply rewarded for your digging and hoeing and planting. The vegetables that you harvest will not only provide Mother Nature's best source of calcium, they will be chock-full of vitamins A and C.

Even the most expensive gourmet specialty shop has nothing that can duplicate the taste of tender young shoots of curly kale that are picked after the first winter frost. And you won't have to travel miles to an Oriental grocery store for bok choy, you can pick some in your garden.

The following pages list a variety of calcium-rich vegetables, each with a brief description, nutrition information, planting instructions, time between planting and harvest, and the names of a few seed companies that offer certain varieties of that vegetable. Although seeds for common vegetables are available in most garden supply outlets throughout the country, many are not available everywhere. The information in this chapter should help you find the seeds you want.

Only a cross-section of seed companies is included. For information on additional seed suppliers, consult the gardening column of your local newspaper, gardening magazines, or books on vegetable gardening. Then you can send for the catalogues of those companies whose seeds you want to plant.

Whether you have an acre of land behind your house, or just a few feet of space behind your apartment, there are some wonderful culinary treats in store for you with the harvest of your high calcium vegetables. Your bones benefit in two ways, from the calcium and other healthful nutrients in the vegetables, and from the exercise you get digging the soil, planting the seeds, cultivating the plants, and harvesting the crops.

Planting High Calcium Vegetables

Following are general guidelines to help you make selections when planning your garden. When sowing seeds, follow specific instructions on individual seed packet. The nutrition information in the listings is for a 1-cup cooked serving, unless otherwise noted; percentages are those of the U.S. RDA. Numbers in parentheses indicate days from planting to harvest. Addresses of seed companies are listed at the end of the chapter.

PLANTING SUMMARY

VEGETABLE	PLANTING DAYS TO MATURITY	DEPTH TO PLANT	DISTANCE BETWEEN ROWS
Beets (for greens)	55-80	1/2-1"	14-16"
	Sow seeds thickly when grown for leaves		
Bok Choy	45-47	1/4-1/2"	18-24"
	Prefer cool weather for best growth		
Broccoli	55-80	1/4-1/2"	24-36"
	Best when matures in cool weather		
Chard, Swiss	60	1/2-1"	18-24"
	Thrives in summer		
Collards	65-75	1/4-1/2"	24-30"
	Plant in spring and late summer		
Kale	55-75	1/4-1/2"	18-24"
	Grows best as fall crop		
Mustard Greens	35-50	1/4-1/2"	12-18"
	Make successive plantings		
Mustard Spinach	28-35	1/4-1/2"	12-18"
	Fast growing; highest calcium		
Okra	50-60	1/2"	24-36"
	Pick pods daily when 2-3" long		
Spinach	45-50	1/2"	12-18"
	Cool weather crop		
Spinach, New Zealand	70-80	1"	12-18"
	Lower calcium than regular; higher oxalic acid		
Turnips (for greens)	35-60	1/2-1"	12-15"
	Sow seeds thickly when grown for leaves		

HIGH CALCIUM VEGETABLES
Figures based on 1 cup, cooked and drained, unless otherwise indicated.
Percentages are based on U.S. RDA for each nutrient.

VEGETABLE	CALORIES	CALCIUM	VIT. A	VIT. C	IRON
Beet Greens	40	16%	147%	60%	15%
Broccoli, chopped	46	18%	44%	163%	10%
Bok Choy (*see* Chinese Cabbage)					
Chard, Swiss, chopped	36	10%	110%	53%	22%
Chinese Cabbage, shredded	20	16%	87%	74%	10%
Collards	26	15%	84%	31%	4%
Dandelion Greens, chopped	35	15%	246%	32%	11%
Kale, chopped	41	9%	192%	89%	7%
Kale, Scotch	37	17%	52%	114%	14%
Mustard Greens, chopped	21	10%	85%	59%	5%
Okra, sliced	50	10%	18%	43%	4%
Spinach	41	24%	295%	30%	36%
Swiss Chard (*see* Chard, Swiss)					
Turnip Greens, chopped	29	20%	158%	66%	6%

AMARANTH

Nutrition Information
    Calories: 28
    Calcium: 27%
    Vitamin A: 73%
    Vitamin C: 90%
    Iron: 16%

Also known as Chinese spinach. See *Spinach* for planting information.

BEETS (FOR GREENS)

Nutrition Information

Calories:	40
Calcium:	16%
Vitamin A:	147%
Vitamin C:	60%
Iron:	15%

Beets are an easy crop to grow under most weather conditions, and successive plantings can be made every 3 weeks. Beets give double dividends: tasty nutritious tops with root beets. Water and mulch well in very hot weather.

The following varieties of beets are recommended for their greens:

Albina Vereduna (formerly Snowhite) (55 days). Curled and wavy tender leaf; ice-white root. Available: Thompson & Morgan.

Albino White Beet (50 days). Green tops similar to Golden; good for greens. Available: Stokes.

Burpee's Golden Beet (55 days). Grown primarily for fine-flavored tops; maintains bright green color during cooler weather. Available: Burpee, Park, Stokes.

Crosby Green Top (60 days). Bright glossy green tops in spring, summer, and fall. Dual purpose beet. Available: Harris, Liberty.

Early Wonder (55 days). Tops grow fast, reach 16"-18" height. Deep red early beet. Available: Burpee, Hastings, Meyer, Olds.

Lutz Green Leaf, Winter Keeper (80 days). Excellent for tender greens; glossy green tops with pink midrib. Available: Burpee.

BOK CHOY (see CHINESE CABBAGE)

BROCCOLI

Nutrition Information (serving size: 1 cup, cooked, chopped)

Calories:	46
Calcium:	18%
Vitamin A:	44%
Vitamin C:	163%
Iron:	10%

Broccoli is easy to grow, and many varieties continue to produce side shoots for continued use even after the main head is cut. Plant in early spring for late spring harvest, or in summer for fall harvest, since broccoli is best when it matures in cool weather. For disease prevention, avoid planting in area where cabbage-type crops grew during the previous year.

In addition to those listed below, there are many other varieties of broccoli, including Sprouting Broccoli and Raab types, that are quick-growing and do not produce heads, whose leaves and loose flower heads can be harvested for greens. There is no data from the USDA for nutritional contents of these varieties.

Cleopatra (55 days). For early planting; cold and drought resistant; uniform heads; vigorous side shoots. Available: Park, Stokes.

Dandy Early (90 days). Compact, non-spreading for narrow rows in small gardens; 10-ounce heads. Available: Thompson & Morgan.

Green Comet Hybrid (55 days). Good for home garden. Single head, 6"-7" across, weight about 1 lb. A popular variety. Available: Burpee, Harris, Liberty, Park, Thompson & Morgan.

Green Goliath (55 days). Tightly budded center heads, heavy yields, many side shoots as secondary crop. Available: Burpee, Stokes.

Premium Crop Hybrid (58 days). Good for spring and fall plantings. Uniform 8"-9" heads; productive yield. Available: Burpee, Harris, Hastings, Liberty, Olds, Park, Stokes, Vesey's.

Spartan Early (60 days). Compact plant developed by Michigan Agricultural Research Station; heavy central head, sprouts develop after head is cut. Available: Olds, Stokes.

Waltham 29 (75 days). Recommended for fall crop; broad even heads, side shoots continue until hard frost. Available: Harris, Liberty.

CHARD, SWISS

Nutrition Information (chopped)

Calories:	36
Calcium:	10%
Vitamin A:	110%
Vitamin C:	53%
Iron:	22%

Swiss chard is a variety of beet, with large fleshy leaves. It is easy to grow and produces tender leaves all season. Stands both hot weather and cold, and will even produce greens in spring if it has been partially protected during winter. Stems may be cooked like asparagus. To harvest, cut whole plant back to 2" above soil.

Fordhook Giant (60 days). Leaves crumpled, thick, and dark green; heavy yields; tender greens. Available: Burpee, Meyer.

Large White Rib (60 days). Tender greens; very ornamental with stems in shades of red, orange, purple, yellow, and white. Available: Thompson & Morgan.

Lucullus (60 days). Thick white ribs, crumpled light green leaves. Productive over long period. Available: Hastings, Olds, Park, Thompson & Morgan.

Perpetual (50 days). Early, very productive variety. Smooth dark green leaves with little midrib. Available: Burpee.

Rhubard Chard (60 days). Red rhubarb-like stalk, dark green crumpled leaves; attractive addition to flower garden. Available: Burpee, Liberty, Park, Thompson & Morgan, Vesey's.

Swiss Chard of Geneve (60 days). Very hardy; withstands severe winters. Very large ribs, celery-like stalks. Available: Park.

CHINESE CABBAGE

Nutrition Information

Calories:	20
Calcium:	16%
Vitamin A:	87%
Vitamin C:	74%
Iron:	10%

You have to be persistent to find this vegetable in seed catalogues. Sometimes it is listed under Cabbages and identified as Chinese Mustard Cabbage. (Although it is a type of cabbage, it does not form a head.) Some catalogues list it under Chinese Greens or Chinese Vegetables as Bok Choy, Pak Choy, or Lei Choy (or Choi). It's worth some detective work to find this vegetable because it's versatile, with thick white stalks that can be substituted for celery and green leafy tops that are somewhat like spinach. Do not confuse Chinese Mustard Cabbage with Chinese Celery Cabbage, which contains only a small amount of calcium.

Bok Choy, Pak Choy, Lei Choy (45 days). Easy to grow, slow-bolting type; white celery-like stalks 8"-10" long, with green leaves. Available: Burpee, Harris, Liberty, Park, Stokes, Thompson & Morgan.

Crispy Choy (45 days). Fast maturing, non-heading bunches of stalks, 7"-8" tall. Available: Burpee.

Mustard Cabbage Bok Choy (heavy). Heavier and hardier type, which resembles white Swiss chard; only inner tender leaves and hearts are eaten. Available: Stokes.

COLLARDS

Nutrition Information

Calories:	26
Calcium:	15%
Vitamin A:	84%
Vitamin C:	31%
Iron:	4%

Collards are a member of the cabbage family, even though they do not form a head. A hardy plant that has been a favorite of Southerners for generations, it may be planted in spring to produce through the summer, and planted again in late summer for a fall/winter harvest. A light freeze even improves the flavor.

Champion (75 days). A new Vates type; plants are short-stemmed with thick leaves; vigorous with high yield potential. Avail: Harris, Meyer.

Georgia (60 days). Old standard popular variety; loose cluster of blue-green spoon-shaped leaves; height 2 to 3 feet. Available: Burpee, Hastings, Liberty, Meyer, Olds, Park.

Hicrop F1 Hybrid (72 days). Adaptable to hot dry weather or cool wet season; stands extreme cold in winter. Mild, sweet flavor. Available: Park, Thompson & Morgan.

Vates (75 days). Developed by Virginia Truck Experiment Station; lower growing and more compact than Georgia; thick broad leaves. Available: Burpee, Harris, Liberty, Meyer, Stokes.

DANDELION GREENS

Nutrition Information

Calories:	35
Calcium:	15%
Vitamin A:	246%
Vitamin C:	32%
Iron:	4%

Most of us think of the dandelion as a "pest" plant and buy weed-killers to rid our lawns of its yellow flower. But those who have savored spring dandelion greens speak glowingly of a pleasant zesty flavor that adds color and texture — as well as calcium and vitamins — to salads, soups, or any greens recipe.

Thick-Leaved Dandelion Greens (95 days). Large, thick, dark green leaves. Vigorous, quick growing. Available: Burpee.

KALE

There are two types of kale, with the Scotch varieties containing almost twice as much calcium as regular kale.

Nutrition Information

KALE		SCOTCH KALE	
Calories:	41	Calories:	37
Calcium:	9%	Calcium:	17%
Vitamin A:	192%	Vitamin A:	52%
Vitamin C:	89%	Vitamin C:	114%
Iron:	7%	Iron:	14%

Kale has a milder flavor than collards, and its curly leaves make it an attractive plant to include in a flower bed. It is grown best as a fall crop, with the flavor improving after a light frost. Do not plant where cabbage, broccoli, or brussels sprouts were planted the previous year.

Scotch Varieties (higher calcium)

Green Curled Scotch (55 days). White-ribbed, finely curled, yellowish-green leaves; height 15". Available: Olds, Stokes.

Vates Curled Blue Scotch (68 days). Dwarf spreading kale with blue-green, finely curled leaves; height about 15". Available: Olds, Meyer, Vesey's.

Other Varieties

Cottagers (70 days). Robust vegetable; early spring producer of tender shoots. Available: Thompson & Morgan.

Dwarf Blue Curled Vates (55 days). Standard dwarf, curled; developed at Virginia Truck Experiment Station. Uniform, compact, short-stemmed plants with finely curled bluish-green leaves. Available: Burpee, Harris, Hastings, Liberty, Park.

Dwarf Green Curled (75 days). Prolonged crop period, tolerates wet conditions and poor soil. Available: Thompson & Morgan.

Siberian Improved Dwarf (65 days). Hardy spreading kale; plants 12"-15" high with plume-like leaves, slightly frilled. Available: Burpee, Hastings, Liberty.

MUSTARD GREENS

Nutrition Information

Calories:	21
Calcium:	10%
Vitamin A:	85%
Vitamin C:	59%
Iron:	5%

Florida Broadleaf (50 days). Large, upright plant, early fast-growing variety. Available: Hastings, Meyer, Stokes.

Fordhook Fancy (40 days). Dark green leaves, deeply curled and fringed, curve in ostrich-like plumes; mild flavor, slow to bolt. Avail: Burpee.

Giant Long Standing Southern Curled (60 days). Large, wide curly leaves, bright green. Available: Hastings, Meyer, Olds.

Green Wave (45 days). Deeply frilled, quick-growing, uniform deep green leaf, resists bolting. Available: Harris, Liberty, Meyer, Stokes.

MUSTARD SPINACH or "TENDERGREEN" MUSTARD

Nutrition Information

Calories:	29
Calcium:	28%
Vitamin A:	295%
Vitamin C:	195%
Iron:	8%

Mustard spinach, listed as tendergreen under Mustard Greens or Spinach in the seed catalogues, is the undisputed winner as the vegetable with the highest calcium content. In addition, mustard spinach has more vitamin A and vitamin C than most high-potency vitamin supplement pills. It's a fast-growing, hardy plant that will turn your garden into a calcium factory.

Tendergreen (28-35 days). Tender, broad, dark green leaves with spinach-like flavor; ribs thin and cream-colored; quick-growing, resistant to heat and drought. Available: Burpee, Harris, Hastings, Meyer, Olds, Park.

OKRA

Nutrition Information

Calories:	50
Calcium:	10%
Vitamin A:	18%
Vitamin C:	44%
Iron:	4%

Okra is the essential ingredient for flavoring and thickening gumbos and other soups. Home-grown okra is a unique taste treat if the pods are picked when they are young and tender.

Clemson Spineless (56 days). Abundant growth, dark green, slightly grooved spineless pods. Grows to 4 feet. Pods best picked when 2"-3" long. Available: Burpee, Hastings, Meyer, Olds, Park.

Dwarf Green Long Pod (52 days). Ribbed pods, dark green, fleshy. Plants grow to height of 2 to 2 1/2 feet. Available: Burpee, Hastings, Meyer.

Emerald (58 days). Dark green spineless pod variety developed by the Campbell Soup Company; plants are highly productive and may grow to 6 foot height. Available: Burpee, Harris.

Lee (50 days). Good in limited space gardens; dark green, nearly spineless pods; plants grow to height of 3 feet. Available: Hastings, Park.

SPINACH

Nutrition Information

Calories:	41
Calcium:	24%
Vitamin A:	295%
Vitamin C:	30%
Iron:	36%

Spinach is a winner for nutrients. Its calcium content is highest of the popular vegetables and it is bursting with vitamin A and iron. Gardeners advise bolting-resistant (long-standing varieties) for spring planting as soon as the soil can be worked, and fall plantings about a month from the average frost date. There are two varieties: savoy type with crinkled leaves, and a smooth-leaf type.

Recommended for Spring Planting

America (50 days). Savoy, glossy, dark green leaves. Heavy yielder, slow bolting. Available: Burpee, Stokes.

Long Standing Bloomsdale (48 days). Heavy yield, savoy dark green leaves, thick texture; very hardy. Available: Burpee, Hastings, Meyer, Olds, Park, Stokes.

Winter Bloomsdale (45 days). Smooth leaf. Plant in early spring or for fall sowing to "winter over" for early spring crop; slow bolting and exceptionally hardy. Available: Burpee, Harris, Liberty.

Other Varieties

Amaranth (Chinese Spinach) (45 days). This type of spinach has a taste of horseradish; tender flavored leaves all summer. Grows to height of 2 to 3 feet. One of the highest calcium vegetables, but contains more oxalic acid than spinach. Available: Thompson & Morgan.

Melody Hybrid (42 days). Good disease resistance; vigorous and fast-growing; popular for home gardens. Available: Burpee, Harris, Liberty, Meyer, Stokes, Thompson & Morgan

Monoppa (45 days). Unique spinach with mellow flavor and low oxalic acid; bolt resistant and winter hardy. Available: Thompson & Morgan.

New Zealand Spinach (70 days). This is not a true spinach, though it has fleshy spinach-like leaves. Gardeners plant it as a summer spinach substitute since it thrives in warm weather. Lower in calcium and higher in oxalic acid than regular spinach. Available: Burpee, Harris, Liberty, Meyer, Park, Stokes, Thompson & Morgan.

Popeye's Choice (50 days). Abundant production; hybrid variety that will stand for prolonged periods without bolting. Available: Vesey's.

TURNIPS (FOR GREENS)

Nutrition Information

Calories:	29
Calcium:	20%
Vitamin A:	158%
Vitamin C:	66%
Iron:	6%

Turnips grow best during cool weather; they may be planted in spring, then again in late summer for a fall crop. Harvest tops for greens while they're young and tender.

Just Right Hybrid (60 days). Heavy cut leaves good for greens; roots white, flattened globe-shaped. Available: Hastings, Park.

Purple Top White Globe (55 days). Popular variety good for early summer harvesting; roots purplish red on upper part and creamy white below. Available: Burpee, Hastings, Liberty, Meyer, Olds, Park, Stokes.

Seven Top (45 days). Grown only for greens (roots are inedible). Cut leaf, very dark green; grows to height of 20"-22". Available: Liberty, Park.

Shoigoin (30 days for foliage, 70 days for roots). Tender mild tops; white globe-shaped roots. Best variety for commercially grown greens. Available: Stokes.

Tokyo Cross Hybrid (35 days). High quality tops for greens; disease resistant; turnips grow 6" across; snow-white. Available: Burpee, Hastings, Meyer, Park, Stokes, Thompson & Morgan.

Seed Sources

W. Atlee Burpee Company, Warminster, Pennsylvania 18974

Harris Seeds, Joseph Harris Company, Inc., Moreton Farm, 3670 Buffalo Road, Rochester, New York 14624

H. G. Hastings Company, 434 Marietta Street, PO Box 4274, Atlanta, Georgia

Liberty Seed Company, PO Box 806, New Philadephia, Ohio 44663

Meyer Seed Company, 600 South Caroline Street, Baltimore, Maryland 21231

L. L. Olds Seed Company, PO Box 7790, 2901 Packers Avenue, Madison, Wisconsin 53707

Park Seed Company, Cokesbury Road, Greenwood, South Carolina 29647

Stokes Seeds, Inc., Box 548, Buffalo, New York 14240

Thompson & Morgan, PO Box 1308, Jackson, New Jersey 08527

Vesey's Seeds, Ltd., York, Box 9000, Charlottetown, Prince Edward Island, Canada C1A 8K6

PART III

COOKING THE HIGH CALCIUM, LOW CALORIE WAY

8

CREATIVE
CALCIUM COOKERY

YOU CAN ENJOY creating a high calcium culinary lifestyle. Accept the challenge of brightening family meals with new food combinations: broccoli with tofu, canned salmon with yogurt, or lamb with rhubarb. The recipes here are intended to give you a start. Once you learn to "think calcium," you'll be able to substitute new ingredients and adapt other recipes to add calcium to your meals.

Two important staples for a high calcium cupboard are nonfat instant dry milk and canned evaporated milk, which can be used in soups, sauces, shakes, and desserts. You can save calories without giving up "whipped cream"; just try the recipes for whipped toppings.

If you're not familiar with the unique flavor and crisp texture of vegetable "greens," it's time to get acquainted. Try bok choy, not only in Chinese stir-fry, but in soups and salads. Substitute figs for raisins. Make your tuna recipes with canned salmon instead (mashing the bones with a fork). Substitute chunks of sardines, with bones, for the turkey in Julienne salads. Make your own salad dressings with buttermilk, tofu, or nonfat yogurt, instead of oil.

"Cream" Sauces and "Cream" Soups

Cream sauces and soups are a good source of calcium, and hardly anyone will suspect if you lower calories by using skim milk. You can add grated cheese to a basic cream sauce for a Sauce Mornay — to turn ordinary noodles into a tasty company treat. Add a little sherry wine to a cream sauce and combine with leftover chicken for an elegant Chicken a la King.

107

Greens

Full of important vitamins, these low calorie vegetables are also a rich source of calcium. Countless recipes exist for broccoli and spinach, but do you know what to do with beet greens, mustard greens, turnip greens, dandelion greens, kale, or collards? (Frozen collard greens, mustard greens, and turnip greens can all substitute for fresh.) Once you've sampled the different varieties of greens, you'll recognize their adaptability for many vegetable recipes.

Tofu

Tofu is an excellent source of protein. It is low in calories, cholesterol, and sodium. Versatile for cooking, it can be baked, fried, or steamed. It is a good calcium source (only if it is coagulated with calcium sulfate or calcium chloride).

With a smooth consistency somewhat between a baked custard and a soft cheese, tofu is difficult to describe to someone who is not familiar with it. Fresh from the container, it tastes bland, but it magically takes on the flavor of any ingredient with which it is combined. When soaked in soy sauce marinade, it tastes like Oriental chicken. Brushed with barbecue sauce and baked in the oven, it tastes like barbecued ribs.

You can spice up salads with pickled tofu cubes, made by marinating them in the juice left in a jar of dill pickles or pickled beets after their contents have been eaten, or in your favorite salad dressing. For fruit salads, marinate the cubes in fruit juice or the syrup from canned fruit. You can float tofu cubes in clear soups. You can crumble it and fry in margarine for low-cholesterol scrambled eggs. The uses for tofu in cooking are practically unlimited.

To keep tofu fresh, pour out the liquid from the package as soon as you open it, and replace with cold water to cover. Replace the water every day, although this will wash out some of the calcium each time. Although you may keep tofu in it's original container, it will stay fresh longer in a larger container that holds more water. Tofu should be eaten within a week of opening.

When a recipe calls for crumbled tofu, place it in a linen tea towel;

twist the ends and gently squeeze out the water. Then crumble it with your fingers. To slice or cube tofu easily, drain it for about an hour in a colander. Lessen draining time by cutting the tofu cake in half or by lining the colander with paper towels and changing them as they get wet.

Frozen tofu. Tofu may be frozen. Freezing changes its appearance and texture: the color changes from creamy white to beige, and the texture become spongy. When thawed tofu is crumbled and fried in cooking oil or margarine, its texture is similar to that of ground beef, and it is popular with vegetarians as a meat substitute. Thawed frozen tofu soaks up marinade more quickly than fresh tofu.

To freeze tofu, cut a 1-pound cake into four pieces. Drain on several thicknesses of paper towels for about five minutes and pat dry. Wrap in freezer wrap or foil and place in freezer for at least 24 hours. To thaw, unwrap and and cover with boiling water for ten minutes. Then drain. To crumble, squeeze gently in the palms of your hands or in a kitchen towel.

Yogurt

Yogurt is one of the most versatile high calcium foods, as it can be eaten right out of the carton as a snack or used as a low calorie substitute for sour cream and mayonnaise. Use it as a base for cold summer soups and breakfast "shakes." Make salad dressings with yogurt instead of oil. Dieters and cholesterol-watchers prefer nonfat yogurt; lowfat yogurt offers a wider variety of flavors.

When cooking with yogurt, don't heat it alone or it may curdle. Instead, combine room temperature yogurt with eggs, flour, or cornstarch before adding to hot foods. Or add the yogurt toward the end of the cooking time by stirring it into the other ingredients with a wire whisk, and then warm over low heat, but *do not bring to a boil.*

DISCOVER YOGURT CREAM CHEESE!

If you've been avoiding eating cream cheese because it's high in fat and calories, try making your own yogurt cream cheese. It looks and tastes like commercial cream cheese, but it has fewer calories, more calcium, and *no fat*, if it is made with nonfat yogurt. Use it instead of butter or margarine on your morning toast or bagel, for cracker spreads and dips, to top a baked potato, for sandwich fillings, or to make a fruit parfait. Try some of the recipes that include yogurt cream cheese as an important ingredient.

It's easy to make yogurt cream cheese in your own kitchen by draining the whey (the liquid) from a carton of yogurt *that contains no gelatin*. Use plain nonfat or low fat yogurt, or flavored yogurt without pieces of fruit.

The consistency of the yogurt cream cheese is determined by the length of time the yogurt drains: the longer the draining period, the thicker the cheese. If you desire the consistency of cream cheese, drain the yogurt overnight, or for 12 to 14 hours (up to 20 hours). If you want a low calorie substitute for sour cream, drain the yogurt for only 3 or 4 hours.

Since the yield of yogurt cheese after draining is approximately half the amount of yogurt in the carton, a 16-ounce carton of yogurt should be used to make 8 ounces of yogurt cream cheese, and an 8-ounce carton to make 4 ounces of yogurt cream cheese.

How to make yogurt cream cheese

There are two options available as methods for draining the yogurt. You can make a bag out of cheesecloth, or you can use a unique new "funnel," which was specially designed for this purpose. Called the *Really Creamy Yogurt Cheese Funnel*, it is convenient, reusable, and easy to clean.

Yogurt cream cheese made from nonfat yogurt has no fat in it. Just one ounce of commercial cream cheese contains a hefty 10 grams of fat, 100 calories, and only 2 percent calcium.

The nutritional content of yogurt cream cheese is variable, depending on the brand and type of yogurt used, the method of draining, and the length of draining time. However, yogurt cream cheese, when made from nonfat yogurt, contains absolutely no fat. Whether made from nonfat or low fat yogurt, yogurt cream cheese contains more calcium, less fat, and fewer calories per ounce than commercial cream cheese.

The following data on the calorie and calcium content of yogurt cream cheese were provided by Triad Publishing Company from nutritional analyses made by an independent laboratory. The samples of yogurt cream cheese came from the Really Creamy Yogurt Cheese Funnel, using Dannon nonfat and plain lowfat yogurt.

These laboratory results indicated that samples ranged between 5 and 7 percent of the U.S. RDA for calcium in one ounce, with yogurt cream cheese made from nonfat yogurt containing no fat and 20 calories, and yogurt cream cheese made from plain low fat yogurt containing 1 gram of fat and 28 calories.

The yogurt cream cheese used in the recipes was prepared with the Really Creamy Yogurt Cheese Funnel, and these data were used in calculating the approximate calorie and calcium contents of the recipes.

Cheesecloth Method. Purchase cheesecloth that is designated for cooking purposes. Cut two lengths of approximately 14 inches. Drape one strip of cheesecloth across a medium-sized bowl and place the other over it at a right angle, so the two pieces are criss-crossed. Run a knife around the inside edge of the yogurt carton. Turn the carton upside down into the bowl.

Gather the four ends together to form a bag. Tie with string or a rubber band. Grasp the tied ends and lift the bag of yogurt several inches up one side of the bowl. Drape the tied ends over the edge of the bowl and secure them in place under the bowl. The yogurt should not touch the whey that drains out.

Refrigerate about 12 hours or overnight. Unfasten the bag and gently transfer the cheese into a storage or serving dish. Keep refrigerated.

How to add yogurt cream cheese to your diet

The more yogurt cream cheese you keep in the refrigerator, the more ways you'll find to use it. Although it can be eaten plain, you can vary the taste with an unlimited number of flavorings, such as jam, maple syrup, honey, brown sugar, fruit juice concentrate, or chopped dried fruit.

If you crave a danish for breakfast, but know you shouldn't, toast an English muffin half, spread it with 1 or 2 ounces of yogurt cream cheese made from nonfat or low fat yogurt, sprinkle with some cinnamon, and toast it under the broiler until it bubbles.

For lunch your options are again unlimited. Make salad and sandwich spreads by combining yogurt cream cheese with salmon or sardines (with bones), chopped vegetables, herbs and spices, or almost any leftovers. As a variation, fill pita bread with salad, raw or marinated vegetables, and yogurt cheese.

For dinner, you can let your imagination run wild. If your favorite cheesecake has a cream cheese base, make it with yogurt cream cheese instead of commercial cream cheese, which is high in calories and has hardly any calcium. Or substitute it for higher-calorie ricotta cheese in lasagna or cheese-filled pasta. Yogurt cream cheese can also be the base for a wide variety of appetizer spreads and dips, and, made from lemon or vanilla-flavored yogurt, makes a calcium-rich and low calorie frosting for cakes and gingerbread.

For your sweet tooth, make bone-building cookies by spreading yogurt cheese on a graham cracker (or between two wafer-type cookies, if you can afford the calories). Vary it by adding chopped dried figs or chopped dates. Flavored yogurt cheese makes a calcium-rich and low calorie frosting for cakes and gingerbread.

The *Really Creamy Yogurt Cheese Funnel* may be ordered directly from Millhopper Marketing, Inc., 1110 Northwest Eighth Avenue, Gainesville, Florida 32601. The cost is $9.95 plus $2 postage and handling.

9
MEAL SUGGESTIONS

YOU MAY want to use the following high calcium menus as a guide for planning your own meals. The menus are offered, not to set arbitrary limits on calorie consumption, but to offer a variety of ways (and calorie levels) to fulfill your calcium requirement. The calorie counts given for each recipe and each meal will help you stay within the calorie level that suits you best. The calcium is given as a percentage of the U.S. RDA. If you are planning a reducing diet, you should consult your physician. You should also consult your physician before increasing the calcium in your diet.

Breakfast Menus

Recipes are given in Chapter 10 for items preceded by a diamond (◊)

1. Total calcium 51% U.S. RDA, total calories 318

FOOD	QTY.	CALORIES	CALCIUM % U.S. RDA
Orange juice (from frozen concentrate)	³/₄ cup	90	2%
Oatmeal (instant Total, regular flavor)	1 packet	100	20%
Skim milk (for cereal)	¹/₂ cup	43	15%
English muffin, toasted	¹/₂	65	7%
Yogurt cream cheese**	1 oz	20	7%

Beverage: for 8 ounces skim milk, add 86 calories and 30% of the U.S. RDA for calcium; coffee or tea contains no calories or calcium (caffeine may interfere with calcium absorption).

** Made from plain nonfat yogurt, drained 12-14 hours

113

2. Total calcium 46% U.S. RDA, total calories 282

FOOD	QTY.	CALORIES	CALCIUM % U.S. RDA
◊ Banana Colada Shake	1 serving	131	28%
◊ Cheese Muffin	1	131	11%
Yogurt cream cheese**	1 oz	20	7%

3. Total calcium 47% U.S. RDA, total calories 327

FOOD	QTY.	CALORIES	CALCIUM % U.S. RDA
Cantaloupe	1/2	95	3%
Whole wheat cereal (Total)	1 cup	100	20%
Skim milk (for cereal)	1/2 cup	43	15%
Whole wheat toast	1 slice	65	2%
Yogurt cream cheese** (on toast)	1 oz	20	7%
Cinnamon (sprinkled on toast)	1/8 tsp	0	*
Sugar (sprinkled on toast)	1/4 tsp	4	*

Beverage: for 8 ounces skim milk, add 86 calories and 30% of the U.S. RDA for calcium; coffee or tea contains no calories or calcium (caffeine may interfere with calcium absorption).

4. Total calcium 32% U.S. RDA, total calories 308

FOOD	QTY.	CALORIES	CALCIUM % U.S. RDA
Orange juice, fresh	3/4 cup	83	2%
English muffin, toasted	1/2	65	7%
Egg, poached (on muffin)	1	80	3%
Mozzarella, part-skim (melted on egg)	1 oz slice	80	20%

Beverage: for 8 ounces skim milk, add 86 calories and 30% of the U.S. RDA for calcium; coffee or tea contains no calories or calcium (caffeine may interfere with calcium absorption).

* Less than 2% U.S. RDA

** Made from plain nonfat yogurt, drained 12-14 hours

5. Total calcium 40% U.S. RDA, total calories 295

FOOD	QTY.	CALORIES	CALCIUM % U.S. RDA
Grapefruit (white)	$^1/_2$	40	*
Waffles, frozen (Aunt Jemima, orig)	2	170	10%
Yogurt cream cheese**	1 oz	20	7%
Maple flavoring (mixed with cheese)	2 drops	0	*
Skim milk	$^3/_4$ cup	65	23%

6. Total calcium 32% U.S. RDA, total calories 290

Orange, sliced	1	60	5%

Open-face sandwich:

Whole wheat toast	1 slice	65	2%
Ham, boiled (slice)	1 oz	65	*
Swiss cheese, natural (slice)	1 oz	100	25%

Beverage: for 8 ounces skim milk, add 86 calories and 30% of the U.S. RDA for calcium; coffee or tea contains no calories or calcium (caffeine may interfere with calcium absorption).

7. Total calcium 47% U.S. RDA, total calories 325

Honeydew melon (6 $^1/_2$" diam)	1/10	45	*
Buckwheat pancakes, 4" (from mix)	3	260	40%
Yogurt cream cheese**	1 oz	20	7%
Maple flavoring (added to cheese)	2 drops	0	*

Beverage: for 8 ounces skim milk, add 86 calories and 30% of the U.S. RDA for calcium; coffee or tea contains no calories or calcium (caffeine may interfere with calcium absorption).

* Less than 2% U.S. RDA

** Nos. 2 and 5: made from plain nonfat yogurt, drained 12-14 hours; no. 3: made from vanilla-flavored low fat yogurt, drained 12-14 hours.

115

Lunch or Dinner Menus

Recipes are given in Chapter 10 for items preceded by a diamond (◊)

1. Total calcium 58% U.S. RDA, total calories 535

FOOD	QTY.	CALORIES	CALCIUM % U.S. RDA
◊ Moussacal	1 serv	362	33%
Shredded lettuce	1 cup	5	*
Tomato	½	13	*
Cucumber (1 ¾" diam.)	4 slices	3	*
◊ Blue Cheese Dressing	1 Tbsp	22	3%
◊ Cocoa Pudding	1 serv	130	22%

Beverage: for 8 ounces skim milk, add 86 calories and 30% of the U.S. RDA for calcium; coffee or tea contains no calories or calcium (caffeine may interfere with calcium absorption).

2. Total calcium 80% U.S. RDA, total calories 500

FOOD	QTY.	CALORIES	CALCIUM % U.S. RDA
◊ Nacho Salmon Pie	1 serv	252	40%
Cooked fresh broccoli, chopped	½ cup	23	9%
Coleslaw:			
Shredded cabbage	½ cup	10	*
Grated carrots	½ cup	15	*
◊ Creamy Yogurt Mayonnaise	2 Tbsp	36	6%
◊ Grammy's Rum Raisin Pudding	1 serv	164	25%

Beverage: for 8 ounces skim milk, add 86 calories and 30% of the U.S. RDA for calcium; coffee or tea contains no calories or calcium (caffeine may interfere with calcium absorption).

* Less than 2% U.S. RDA

** Made from vanilla-flavored low fat yogurt, drained 12-14 hours

3. *Total calcium 62% U.S. RDA, total calories 498*

FOOD	QTY.	CALORIES	CALCIUM % U.S. RDA
◊ Creamy Dilly Scallops	1 serv	271	34%
Chopped spinach (frozen)	3.3 oz	20	10%
Broiled tomato slices:			
Tomato	1	25	*
Parmesan cheese, grated	1 tsp	9	2%
◊ Rhuberry Mousse	1 serv	173	16%

Beverage: for 8 ounces skim milk, add 86 calories and 30% of the U.S. RDA for calcium; coffee or tea contains no calories or calcium (caffeine may interfere with calcium absorption).

4. *Total calcium 44% U.S. RDA, total calories 566*

FOOD	QTY.	CALORIES	CALCIUM % U.S. RDA
◊ Mayapore Lamb	1 serv	332	24%
Rice, brown	¹/₂ cup	115	2%
Beet greens, 1" pieces (steamed, with lemon juice)	¹/₂ cup	20	8%
◊ Pina Colada Sorbet	1 serv	99	10%

Beverage: for 8 ounces skim milk, add 86 calories and 30% of the U.S. RDA for calcium; coffee or tea contains no calories or calcium (caffeine may interfere with calcium absorption).

5. *Total calcium 64% U.S. RDA, total calories 515*

FOOD	QTY.	CALORIES	CALCIUM % U.S. RDA
◊ New England Oyster Chowder	1 serv	213	29%
Oyster crackers	10	30	*
◊ Broccoli Yogur-Tofu Bake	1 serv	177	32%
Cantaloupe (5" diam.)	¹/₂	95	3%

Beverage: for 8 ounces skim milk, add 86 calories and 30% of the U.S. RDA for calcium; coffee or tea contains no calories or calcium (caffeine may interfere with calcium absorption).

* Less than 2% U.S. RDA

6. *Total calcium 52%, total calories 416*

FOOD	QTY.	CALORIES	CALCIUM % U.S. RDA
◊ Buttermilk Gazpacho	1 serv	121	17%
◊ Sardine Muffin Pizza	1 serv	234	35%
Strawberries, whole	¹/₂ cup	23	*
Pineapple, diced	¹/₂ cup	38	*

Beverage: for 8 ounces skim milk, add 86 calories and 30% of the U.S. RDA for calcium; coffee or tea contains no calories or calcium (caffeine may interfere with calcium absorption).

7. *Total calcium 65% U.S. RDA, total calories 526*

◊ Chicken Ricotini	1 serving	283	34%
◊ Hawaiian Carrot Salad	1 serving	85	11%
Swiss chard, chopped (steamed)	¹/₂ cup	18	5%
Butterscotch pudding (Jell-O) made with skim milk	¹/₂ cup	140	15%

Beverage: for 8 ounces skim milk, add 86 calories and 30% of the U.S. RDA for calcium; coffee or tea contains no calories or calcium (caffeine may interfere with calcium absorption).

* Less than 2% U.S. RDA

10
RECIPES

Appetizers

Blue Cheese Spread

1 ounce blue cheese
Yogurt cream cheese made from 8 ounces plain nonfat yogurt*
2 tablespoons chopped parsley
Few drops Worcestershire sauce

Mash blue cheese with a fork. Combine with remaining ingredients. Refrigerate for a few hours. Good for stuffing celery or filling a Yogurt Cheezapple *(see recipe)*. Makes about $1/2$ cup.

Calcium (1 oz): 10% U.S. RDA
Calories (1 oz): 45

Herbed Yogurt Cream Cheese

Yogurt cream cheese made from 8 ounces plain nonfat yogurt*
1 clove garlic, minced
1 teaspoon chopped parsley
1 teaspoon chopped chives
1 teaspoon fresh chopped dill (or $1/2$ tsp dried)
$1/4$ teaspoon salt

Combine all ingredients; refrigerate several hours. Makes about $1/2$ cup.

Calcium (1 oz): 7% U.S. RDA
Calories (1 oz): 26

* Drain yogurt 12-14 hours.

Creamy Cucumber Canapes

1 clove garlic
Yogurt cream cheese made from 8 ounces plain nonfat yogurt*
1 teaspoon chopped fresh dill (or $1/2$ teaspoon dried)
$1/4$ teaspoon chopped chives
$1/4$ teaspoon basil
8 slices unpeeled cucumber, $1/4$" thick
2 radishes, thinly sliced

Drop garlic into small amount of boiling water for 1 minute; crush. Combine garlic, yogurt cream cheese, dill, chives, and basil. Refrigerate for several hours or overnight.

Dry cucumber slices with paper towels. Mound with cheese mixture and top each with a radish slice. Chill before serving. Serves 4.

Calcium per serving: 7% U.S. RDA
Calories per serving: 35

Salmon Tofu Spread
Serve as a cracker spread, sandwich filling, or celery stuffing.

1 can (7 $1/2$ oz) salmon, drained
8 ounces tofu (made with calcium sulfate or calcium chloride)**
2 tablespoons lemon juice
$1/3$ cup chopped green onions
1 tablespoon horseradish
2 teaspoons Dijon-style mustard
1 teaspoon chopped fresh dill (or $1/2$ tsp dried)

Remove skin from salmon, but *do not discard bones*. Mash bones and flake salmon with a fork, or use food processor.

Place tofu on a kitchen towel; pull up the ends to make a pouch, then gently twist and squeeze out the water. Combine crumbled tofu with remaining ingredients. Refrigerate. Makes about 2 cups.

Calcium ($1/4$ cup): 10% U.S. RDA
Calories ($1/2$ cup): 69

* Drain yogurt 12-14 hours.
** Calcium content is based on tofu coagulated with calcium sulfate or calcium chloride.

Stuffed Cherry Tomatoes

The filling can also be used as a sandwich filling, cracker spread, or as a stuffing for celery.

18 cherry tomatoes
1 can (3 ³/₄ oz) sardines (with bones), drained
2 tablespoons chopped green onion
2 tablespoons chopped ripe olives
1 tablespoon lemon juice
1 teaspoon horseradish
Yogurt cream cheese made from 8 oz plain nonfat yogurt
    (drained 12 to 14 hours)

Slice tops off tomatoes and use a small teaspoon (or infant feeding spoon) to scoop out seeds and pulp, leaving just the shell. Turn tomatoes upside down on paper towels to drain while you prepare the filling.

Mash sardines or put in food processor for few seconds. Add onion, olives, lemon juice, and horseradish; stir until well blended. Mix in the yogurt cream cheese. Fill the tomatoes.

Refrigerate for several hours before serving. Serves 6.

Calcium per serving: 13% U.S. RDA
Calories per serving: 72

Soups

Broccoli-Bok Choy Bisque

$^3/_4$ pound fresh broccoli (flowerets, leaves, stems)
2 cups bok choy (leaves and stems)
$^3/_4$ cup chopped onion
$^1/_2$ tablespoon margarine
2 cloves garlic, minced
4 cups water
2 chicken bouillon cubes
1 cup cubed parsnips
$^1/_2$ cup cubed potatoes
$^1/_2$ teaspoon curry powder
$^1/_2$ teaspoon celery salt
1 can (12 oz) evaporated skimmed milk
2 carrots, grated

Split broccoli stems and cut into 2-inch pieces. Slice bok choy stems into 1-inch strips. Set aside.

Saute onion in margarine until transparent; add garlic and cook for 2 minutes.

Bring water and bouillon cubes to a boil in a large pot. When bouillon cubes have dissolved, add, onion, broccoli, bok choy stems, parsnips, potatoes, curry powder, and celery salt. Simmer on low heat 15 minutes. Remove from heat.

Remove vegetables from broth and chop coarsely with a knife or put into food processor in small batches. Return to the broth with bok choy leaves, evaporated milk, and grated carrots; simmer 5 minutes. Serve hot.

Serves 6.

Calcium per serving: 28% U.S. RDA
Calories per serving: 140

Buttermilk Gazpacho

$1/2$ cup finely chopped onion
1 tablespoon margarine
3 medium tomatoes, peeled and chopped
1 clove garlic, minced
$1/2$ teaspoon celery salt
1 cucumber, peeled and seeded
$3/4$ cup chopped green pepper
2 cups buttermilk
$1/2$ cup tomato juice
1 tablespoon white vinegar
1 teaspoon Worcestershire sauce
$1/8$ teaspoon cayenne pepper (or chili powder)
Croutons, optional

Saute onion in margarine until transparent. Add tomatoes, garlic, and celery salt and cook on moderate heat 3-4 minutes.

Chop cucumber and green pepper coarsely (may use food processor). Combine with tomato mixture. Add remaining ingredients and mix well. Refrigerate. Serve chilled, with croutons (not included in calcium/calorie count).

Serves 4.

Calcium per serving: 17% U.S. RDA
Calories per serving: 121

Grammy's Borscht

3 medium potatoes
1 teaspoon salt
1 package (10 oz) frozen chopped spinach
1 pound fresh rhubarb, diced (or frozen rhubarb, thawed)
5 tablespoons lemon juice
$1/3$ cup sugar
2 eggs
1 cup evaporated skimmed milk
1 cup skim milk
Nonfat yogurt, optional

Peel and quarter potatoes. Bring 6 cups salted water to a boil in large pot; add potatoes and cook 10 minutes. Add spinach, rhubarb, lemon juice, and sugar; cook over medium heat 20 minutes. Remove from heat and let cool.

Beat eggs with a wire whisk or rotary beater. Cook the 2 cups of milk over moderate heat until very hot, then add very gradually to eggs, beating continuously with a wire whisk as you pour. Cool about 15 minutes.

Add spinach mixture to egg mixture, beating continuously. Refrigerate until very cold.

To serve, top with a spoonful of nonfat yogurt (not included in calorie/calcium count).

Serves 8.

Calcium per serving: 23% U.S. RDA
Calories per serving: 138

New England Oyster Chowder

3 medium potatoes, peeled and quartered
1 pound raw oysters, in "liquor"
1 leek, white part only, chopped
2 carrots, grated
$^1/_2$ cup chopped celery
$^1/_2$ teaspoon celery salt
2 tablespoons margarine
2 tablespoons flour
4 cups skim milk
$^1/_4$ teaspoon pepper
Chopped parsley garnish

Place potatoes in boiling salted water to cover and cook for about 10 minutes, until easily pierced with a fork. Drain. Cut into cubes.

Drain oyster liquor into a saucepan; add chopped leek and simmer on low heat for about 5 minutes, stirring a few times. Add carrots, celery, and celery salt; cover pan and cook for about 3 minutes. Add potatoes.

Melt margarine in a saucepan and gradually stir in flour with a wire whisk until well blended. Add milk and pepper, and cook on moderate heat, stirring constantly, until mixture thickens and comes to a boil. Lower heat.

Add vegetables and simmer for about 5 minutes, stirring occasionally. Coarsely chop the oysters, then add to mixture and simmer 5 minutes. To serve, sprinkle with chopped parsley.

Serves 6.

Calcium per serving: 29% U.S. RDA
Calories per serving: 213

Rhubarb Summer Soup

1 pound fresh rhubarb, diced (or 16 oz unsweetened frozen rhubarb)
$^3/_4$ cup orange juice
4 tablespoons sugar
$1^1/_2$ cups buttermilk
$^1/_2$ cup plain nonfat yogurt
$^1/_8$ teaspoon nutmeg

Combine rhubarb, orange juice, and sugar in a saucepan and cook on moderate heat for about 15 minutes, until rhubarb is tender. Remove from heat and let cool.

Add buttermilk, yogurt, and nutmeg, and stir until well blended. Refrigerate several hours before serving.

Serves 4.

Calcium per serving: 26% U.S. RDA
Calories per serving: 140

Salads

Pineapple Cream Cheese Salad

Yogurt cream cheese (made from 8 oz plain nonfat yogurt,
    drained 12-14 hrs)
1 can (8 oz) unsweetened sliced pineapple
1 tablespoon chopped almonds
1 teaspoon pineapple preserves
Shredded lettuce

Combine yogurt cream cheese, almonds, and preserves. Refrigerate for several hours to stiffen.

With a teaspoon, form into small balls. Place over pineapple slices on shredded lettuce. Serves 4.

Calcium per serving: 12% U.S. RDA
Calories per serving: 96

Apple-Fig Salad

Yogurt cream cheese (made from 8 oz vanilla-flavored yogurt,
    drained 12-14 hrs)
2 tablespoons apple juice frozen concentrate (thawed)
2 tablespoons nonfat instant dry milk
$1/2$ cup chopped celery
2 apples, peeled and diced
3 Calimyrna figs, chopped
1 tablespoon chopped almonds, optional
Shredded lettuce

Combine yogurt cream cheese, apple juice concentrate, and milk. Stir in remaining ingredients. Refrigerate for several hours. Serve on shredded lettuce.

Serves 4.

Calcium per serving: 11% U.S. RDA
Calories per serving: 129 (142 with almonds)

Hawaiian Carrot Salad

8 ounces tofu (made with calcium sulfate or calcium chloride)
2 tablespoons lemon juice
$1/4$ teaspoon coriander
$1/8$ teaspoon curry powder
1 cup grated carrots
$1/2$ cup chopped celery
2 tablespoons shredded coconut
$1/2$ cup unsweetened pineapple tidbits
6 ounces pineapple-flavored yogurt
Shredded lettuce

Place tofu on a linen kitchen towel; pull up the ends to make a pouch, and gently twist and squeeze out the water. Crumble tofu into blender or food processor; add lemon juice and spices; process 15 seconds. Combine with carrots, celery, coconut, pineapple, and yogurt. Refrigerate.

Serve on shredded lettuce. Serves 6.

Calcium per serving: 11% U.S. RDA
Calories per serving: 85

Scallop-Artichoke Salad

1 pound fresh bay scallops, with "liquor"
2 tablespoons dry vermouth
8 ounces plain nonfat yogurt
2 teaspoons horseradish
1 teaspoon Worcestershire sauce
1 tablespoon lemon juice
1 teaspoon chopped fresh dill (or $^1/_2$ tsp dried)
$^1/_3$ cup chopped green onions
1 jar (6 oz) marinated artichoke hearts, drained and sliced
Shredded lettuce

Trim white muscle from scallops. Drain liquor into frying pan; add vermouth and bring to a boil. Reduce heat and add scallops; cover and poach 5 minutes. Remove from heat and let cool.

Combine yogurt, horseradish, Worcestershire sauce, lemon juice, and dill. Mix in green onions, artichoke hearts, and scallops. Refrigerate several hours. Serve on shredded lettuce.

Serves 4.

Calcium per serving: 26% U.S. RDA
Calories per serving: 220

Salad Dressings

Blue Cheese Dressing

$^1/_2$ cup plain nonfat yogurt
1 ounce blue cheese
$^1/_4$ teaspoon celery salt
Dash Worcestershire sauce

Combine all ingredients. Refrigerate.

Makes about $^1/_2$ cup.

Calcium (1 Tbsp): 3% U.S. RDA
Calories (1 Tbsp): 22

Parmesano Dressing

$^1/_2$ cup plain nonfat yogurt
1 clove garlic, minced
1 tablespoon Parmesan cheese
1 tablespoon chives
$^1/_2$ teaspoon basil
$^1/_4$ teaspoon oregano

Combine all ingredients. Refrigerate. Makes about $^2/_3$ cup.

Calcium (1 Tbsp): 3% U.S. RDA
Calories (1 Tbsp): 15

Thousand Island Dressing

$^1/_2$ cup plain nonfat yogurt
2 tablespoons chili sauce
2 tablespoons sweet pickle relish
$^1/_2$ teaspoon horseradish
Chopped white from 1 hard-boiled egg

Combine all ingredients. Refrigerate. Makes about $^3/_4$ cup.

Calcium (1 Tbsp): 3% U.S. RDA
Calories (1 Tbsp): 17

Creamy Yogurt Mayonnaise

$^1/_2$ cup plain nonfat yogurt
2 teaspoons lemon juice
1 teaspoon sugar
1 teaspoon Dijon-style mustard
$^1/_4$ teaspoon salt
$^1/_8$ teaspoon coriander, optional
$^1/_8$ teaspoon paprika

Combine all ingredients. Refrigerate. Makes about 2/3 cup.

Calcium (1 Tbsp): 3% U.S. RDA
Calories (1 Tbsp): 18

Cucumber-Yogurt Dressing

1 cucumber, peeled and seeded
$^1/_2$ cup plain nonfat yogurt
2 tablespoons chopped green onions
2 tablespoons chopped parsley
2 tablespoons buttermilk
2 tablespoons vinegar
1 teaspoon chopped fresh dill (or $^1/_2$ tsp dried)
$^1/_4$ teaspoon salt
$^1/_4$ teaspoon pepper

Chop cucumber coarsely. Combine with remaining ingredients and stir until blended. Refrigerate until chilled.

Makes about $1^1/_2$ cups.

Calories (1 Tbsp): 14
Calcium (1 Tbsp): 3% U.S. RDA

Oriental Tofu Dressing

8 ounces tofu (made with calcium sulfate or calcium chloride)
$^1/_3$ cup buttermilk
3 tablespoons frozen pineapple juice concentrate (thawed)
2 tablespoons lemon juice
$1^1/_2$ tablespoons light soy sauce
1 tablespoon cider vinegar
2 cloves garlic, minced

Place tofu in linen kitchen towel; pull up the ends to make a pouch, and gently twist and squeeze out the water. Crumble the tofu into a food processor or blender; add remaining ingredients and process 30 seconds or until smooth.

Makes about 1 cup.

Calcium (1 Tbsp): 3% U.S. RDA
Calories (1 Tbsp): 14

Entrees

Nacho Salmon Pie

$^1/_2$ tablespoon soft margarine
$^1/_2$ cup cheese cracker crumbs (about 2 oz)
1 can (15 $^1/_2$ oz) salmon
$^1/_2$ cup plain nonfat yogurt
1 can (4 oz) mild or hot chili peppers, chopped
$^1/_3$ cup chopped green onions
1 ounce sliced ripe olives
1 tablespoon lemon juice
1 teaspoon Dijon-type mustard
3 eggs
1 cup evaporated skimmed milk, undiluted
4 ounces Swiss cheese, grated

Preheat oven to 375 degrees.

Grease bottom and sides of a 9-inch pie plate with the margarine. Sprinkle with cracker crumbs, reserving 2 tablespoons.

Drain salmon and remove the skin, but do not discard the bones. Flake the salmon and mash the bones with a fork, or mix in food processor for about 30 seconds. Combine with yogurt, chili peppers, onions, olives, lemon juice, and mustard.

Beat eggs and milk with wire whisk; mix in grated cheese. Add to salmon mixture. Stir thoroughly, and pour into pie plate. Sprinkle with remaining cracker crumbs. Bake 35 minutes, until top is lightly browned. Serve hot or cold.

Serves 8.

Calcium per serving: 40% U.S. RDA
Calories per serving: 252

Cancun Chicken Enchiladas

4 whole chicken breasts
2 stalks celery, chopped
1 carrot, cut into 4 pieces
$^1/_2$ teaspoon salt, or to taste
$^3/_4$ cup chopped onion
1 tablespoon margarine
1 can (28 oz) whole tomatoes
$^1/_2$ cup chopped green pepper
2 cloves garlic, crushed
2 tablespoons tomato paste
1 teaspoon sugar
$^1/_2$ teaspoon salt, or to taste
$^1/_8$ teaspoon thyme
8 corn tortillas (soft)
Yogurt cream cheese (made from 24 oz plain nonfat yogurt,
     drained 12-14 hrs)
1 can (4 oz) chili peppers, chopped
8 ounces Monterey Jack cheese, grated

Place chicken breasts, celery, and carrot in saucepan. Add salt. Add water to cover, and simmer for about 40 minutes, until chicken is tender. Drain chicken and refrigerate.

Saute onion in margarine until transparent. Add tomatoes, green pepper, garlic, tomato paste, seasonings, and $^1/_3$ cup water. Simmer 15 minutes on moderate heat; lower heat.

Brown tortillas lightly in a frying pan (non-stick preferred) for about 1 minute on each side; cover with foil and keep warm in oven until all are browned. Shred chicken with 2 forks.

Preheat oven to 350 degrees. Spread a few spoonfuls of tomato sauce over the bottom of a baking pan. Divide yogurt cream cheese into 8 parts and spread one portion across the center third of each tortilla. Cover with shredded chicken, 1 tablespoon of tomato sauce, and a sprinkle of chopped chiles. Fold over from both sides, and place seam side down in pan. Cover with tomato sauce and sprinkle with grated cheese. Bake 30 minutes. Serves 8.

Calcium per serving: 41% U.S. RDA
Calories per serving: 368

Chicken Ricotini

2 whole chicken breasts
1 package (10 oz) frozen chopped spinach
$1/2$ cup part skim ricotta cheese
3 tablespoons Parmesan cheese
3 tablespoons plain nonfat yogurt
2 cloves garlic, minced
1 can (6 oz) tomato paste
1 cup water
$1/2$ teaspoon basil
$1/4$ teaspoon oregano
$1/2$ teaspoon sugar
2 ounces mozzarella cheese, grated

Preheat oven to 350 degrees. Skin and bone chicken breasts and cut in half to make 4 fillets. Place each fillet between 2 sheets of wax paper, and pound lightly to flatten.

Cook spinach according to package directions. Drain. Mix spinach with ricotta cheese, Parmesan cheese, yogurt, and 1 clove minced garlic. Place one-fourth of the spinach mixture in the center of each chicken breast; roll to enclose. Place in greased baking pan, seam side down. Bake, uncovered, 30 minutes.

Combine tomato paste, water, basil, oregano, sugar, and remaining garlic in a small saucepan and cook on low heat 5 minutes. Pour over chicken. Sprinkle chicken with mozzarella cheese. Return to oven for 5 to 10 minutes and heat, uncovered, until cheese melts.

Serves 4.

Calcium per serving: 34% U.S. RDA
Calories per serving: 283

Singapore Shrimp

1 can (20 oz) unsweetened pineapple tidbits
3 tablespoons brown sugar, tightly packed
2 tablespoons cornstarch
2 tablespoons white vinegar
2 tablespoons light soy sauce
1-inch piece fresh ginger, peeled and chopped (about 1 Tbsp)
1 tablespoon margarine
2 cloves garlic, minced
1 pound fresh shrimp, peeled and deveined
$2^1/_2$ cups shredded bok choy
$^1/_2$ cup chopped green onions

Drain pineapple, reserving the juice. Set aside $^1/_4$ cup pineapple juice. Combine remaining pineapple juice, brown sugar, cornstarch, vinegar, and soy sauce in a saucepan; stir until blended. Cook on low heat until mixture thickens. Add ginger and pineapple; simmer 3 minutes. Remove from heat.

Melt margarine in frying pan and saute garlic until lightly browned. Add shrimp and saute on each side until shrimp turn pink. Add to pineapple mixture.

In the same frying pan, cook bok choy, green onions, and reserved pineapple juice on low heat until bok choy wilts, about 3 minutes. Add to pineapple-shrimp mixture and heat thoroughly. Serve with rice.

Serves 4.

Calcium per serving: 21% U.S. RDA
Calories per serving: 318

Creamy-Dilly Scallops

1 pound bay or sea scallops, with "liquor"
$^1/_2$ cup chopped green onions
$^3/_4$ cup dry white wine
$1^1/_2$ tablespoons margarine
$1^1/_2$ tablespoons flour
1 cup evaporated skim milk, undiluted
1 teaspoon fresh chopped dill (or $^1/_2$ tsp dried)

Drain liquor from scallops into a saucepan. Remove white muscle from scallops.

Add chopped green onions to scallop liquor and simmer on low heat for a few minutes; add wine and return to a simmer. Add scallops, cover, and simmer until tender, about 5 minutes for sea scallops, 3-4 minutes for bay scallops.

In another saucepan, melt margarine and gradually stir in flour with a wire whisk until well blended. Add milk slowly, stirring until sauce thickens. Add scallop mixture and dill. Heat thoroughly. Serve over rice or pasta.

Serves 4.

Calcium per serving: 34% U.S. RDA
Calories per serving: 271

Mayapore Lamb

1^1/2 pounds boneless lamb shoulder
^{1}/2 teaspoon salt, or to taste
^{3}/4 cup chopped onion
1 tablespoon oil
^{1}/2 cup chopped celery
1 apple, diced
^{1}/2 cup apple juice
2 tablespoons lemon juice
^{1}/2 teaspoon cinnamon
1 pound fresh rhubarb, diced (or unsweetened frozen)
3 tablespoons sugar
8 ounces plain nonfat yogurt

Trim fat off lamb; cut into cubes. Sprinkle with salt.

Saute onion in oil until transparent. Push onion to edge of pan and add lamb cubes. Saute over moderate heat until meat is lightly browned. Add celery, apple, apple juice, lemon juice, and cinnamon. Cover and simmer for about 30 minutes, until lamb is tender.

Add rhubarb and sugar. Simmer, covered, 10-15 minutes, until rhubarb is fully cooked. Take pan off heat and remove cover; let cool for about 15 minutes. Stir in yogurt. Just before serving, warm on low heat; do not bring to a boil.

Serves 4.

Calcium per serving: 25% U.S. RDA
Calories per serving: 325

Moussacal

3/4 cup chopped onion
1 tablespoon oil
1 1/2 pounds ground beef
1 can (28 oz) tomatoes
1/3 cup red wine
2 cloves garlic, minced
3 tablespoons tomato paste
1/2 teaspoon cinnamon
1 2-pound eggplant, peeled and sliced
2/3 cup buttermilk
1/3 cup bread crumbs
1/2 cup Parmesan cheese
15 ounces part-skim ricotta cheese
8 ounces plain nonfat yogurt
1/2 teaspoon nutmeg
3 eggs, beaten well
2 tablespoons margarine
2 tablespoons flour
2 cups skim milk

Saute onion in oil on moderate heat until lightly browned. Add meat and cook until well browned. Add tomatoes, wine, garlic, tomato paste, and cinnamon. Simmer on low heat 15 minutes.

Dip eggplant slices into buttermilk and place on cookie sheet in one layer. Place under preheated broiler until lightly browned.

Preheat oven to 350 degrees. Sprinkle a third of the bread crumbs on the bottom of a 9" x 13" baking pan. Cover with single layer of eggplant slices. Cover eggplant with meat sauce, and sprinkle with bread crumbs and Parmesan. Add second layer of eggplant, meat sauce, crumbs and Parmesan.

Combine ricotta cheese, yogurt, and nutmeg. Add beaten eggs.

Heat margarine until it starts to bubble; add flour gradually with a wire whisk and mix well. Heat milk almost to boiling point and add slowly, stirring constantly with wire whisk until mixture thickens. Add slowly to ricotta mixture, stirring constantly with a wire whisk. Pour over eggplant.

Bake 1 hour. To serve, cut into squares. Serves 10.

Calcium per serving: 33% U.S. RDA
Calories per serving: 360

Salmon Strata

14 slices soft white bread, crusts removed
1 can (15 $\frac{1}{2}$ oz) salmon (with bones), drained
Yogurt cream cheese (made from 16 oz plain nonfat yogurt,
   drained 12-14 hrs)
4 tablespoons grated Parmesan cheese
$\frac{1}{4}$ cup finely chopped green onions
1 teaspoon Dijon-style mustard
1 teaspoon soft margarine
7 eggs
3 $\frac{1}{2}$ cups skim milk

Prepare a day ahead, or at least 8 hours before serving.

Remove skin from salmon, but do not discard bones. Mash bones and flake salmon with a fork, or mix with food processor for 30 seconds. Combine with yogurt cream cheese, Parmesan cheese, green onions, and mustard.

Grease a 9" x 13" baking pan with the margarine. Place half the bread slices in the pan in one layer. Spread with salmon mixture. Top with remaining bread slices. Beat eggs with skim milk and pour over salmon "sandwiches." Cover pan and place in refrigerator for at least 8 hours.

Preheat oven to 350 degrees. Bake strata uncovered 1 hour, until top is lightly browned. To serve, cut with a serrated knife into 8 portions.

Serves 8.

Calcium per serving: 45% U.S. RDA
Calories per serving: 360

Broccoli Yogur-Tofu Bake

1 pound broccoli (flowerets, leaves, stems)
2 tablespoons margarine
2 tablespoons flour
8 ounces plain nonfat yogurt
4 ounces Swiss cheese, grated
2 tablespoons grated Parmesan cheese
$^1/_2$ teaspoon dry mustard
3 eggs
8 ounces tofu (made with calcium sulfate or calcium chloride)

Preheat oven to 350 degrees.

Split broccoli stems and cut into $1^1/_2$-inch pieces. Cook broccoli in salted water for about 10 minutes. Drain. Spread evenly in a greased 10-inch pie plate.

Heat margarine on low heat until it starts to bubble; add flour gradually, mixing well with a wire whisk. Slowly blend in yogurt, stirring constantly with a wire whisk until mixture thickens. Add Swiss cheese, Parmesan cheese, and dry mustard; continue stirring until cheese is melted. Remove from heat.

Beat eggs with a wire whisk. As you beat, gradually add a small amount of cheese sauce to the eggs. Add the remaining sauce and mix thoroughly.

Place tofu on a linen kitchen towel; pull up the ends to make a pouch, and then gently twist and squeeze out the water. Mix crumbled tofu into the cheese sauce and whisk vigorously. Pour over broccoli.

Bake about 30 minutes or until top is lightly browned. Cut into wedges.

Serves 8.

Calcium per serving: 32% U.S. RDA
Calories per serving: 177

Note: Calcium content is based on tofu coagulated with calcium sulfate or calcium chloride.

Bayou Shrimp Gumbo

1 pound fresh shrimp
1 can (28 oz) tomatoes
3/4 cup chopped onions
1 1/2 tablespoons margarine
2 tablespoons flour
1 bay leaf
1/2 teaspoon celery salt
1/2 teaspoon pepper
1 1/2 teaspoons Worcestershire sauce
1/2 teaspoon ground thyme
1 teaspoon sugar
1 package (10 oz) frozen cut okra
1 cup chopped celery
3/4 cup chopped green pepper

Peel and devein shrimp; rinse with cold water and pat dry with paper towels. Drain tomatoes, reserving about 1/2 cup juice, and cut up.

In a large frying pan, saute onions in margarine on low heat until transparent. Gradually stir in flour with a wire whisk and continue cooking and stirring until flour is very lightly browned. Add reserved juice from tomatoes and stir until mixture is smooth. Add tomatoes, bay leaf, and seasonings; simmer 10 minutes.

Add shrimp, okra, celery, and green pepper and simmer about 5 minutes. Remove bay leaf and serve over rice.

Serves 4.

Calcium per serving: 24% U.S. RDA
Calories per serving: 279

Brocco-Baked Fish

$^3/_4$ pound fresh broccoli (flowerets, leaves, stems)
$^1/_2$ cup part-skim ricotta cheese
4 tablespoons grated Parmesan cheese
1 teaspoon chopped chives
6 fish fillets (approx. $1^1/_2$ pounds sole, scrod, flounder)
$^1/_3$ cup evaporated skimmed milk, undiluted
4 ounces Gruyere cheese, grated

Split broccoli stems and cut into 2-inch pieces. Add broccoli to boiling salted water; cover and cook for about 10 minutes, until just tender. Drain.

Preheat oven to 400 degrees.

Chop broccoli coarsely. Combine with ricotta cheese, Parmesan cheese, and chives. Divide into 6 portions. Spoon one portion onto center of each fillet, rolling to enclose the filling. Place in a lightly greased baking pan seam side down, and bake 15 minutes.

Heat milk until it just comes to a boil; add grated Gruyere and stir constantly until cheese is melted. Pour over fillets and continue baking for an additional 5-8 minutes, until cheese is lightly browned.

Serves 6.

Calcium per serving: 41% of U.S. RDA
Calories per serving: 247

Spinach Lasagne Bolognese

$^1/_2$ pound lasagna noodles (9 strips)
$1^1/_2$ pounds fresh spinach, chopped (or 15 oz frozen, chopped)
$^2/_3$ cup chopped onion
1 tablespoon margarine
1 can (28 oz) tomatoes, cut up
4 tablespoons tomato paste
1 carrot, grated
2 cloves garlic, minced
1 tablespoon sugar
$^1/_2$ teaspoon basil
$^2/_3$ cup evaporated skimmed milk, undiluted
$^1/_2$ cup chopped parsley
1 egg, beaten
$1^1/_2$ cups part-skim ricotta cheese
8 ounces mozzarella, grated
$^1/_2$ cup grated Parmesan cheese

Place noodles in a large pot with at least 6 quarts of boiling, salted water; cook according to package directions. Drain. Rinse with cold water.

Cook spinach in $^1/_2$ cup salted water in covered pot until wilted, about 3-4 minutes (or cook frozen spinach according to package directions). Drain. Chop coarsely.

Saute chopped onion in margarine until transparent. Add tomatoes (including juice), tomato paste, carrot, garlic, sugar, and basil, and simmer 10 minutes, stirring occasionally. Add milk and $^1/_4$ cup chopped parsley and simmer 5 minutes, stirring occasionally.

Combine beaten egg, ricotta, and remaining parsley.

Preheat oven to 350 degrees. Spoon a few tablespoons of tomato sauce over the bottom of a 9" x 13" baking dish. Place three lasagna noodles in the pan. Spread half the spinach mixture over the noodles. Sprinkle with one-third of the Parmesan cheese, one-third of the mozzarella, and one-third of the tomato sauce. Repeat, ending with tomato sauce layer. Bake 35 minutes. Serves 8 to 10.

Calcium per serving: 46% U.S. RDA (8 serv.); 37% (10 serv.)
Calories per serving: 349 (8 serv.); 279 (10 serv.)

Tofu Nuggets Napoli

16 ounces tofu (made with calcium sulfate or calcium chloride)
1 can (8 oz) tomato sauce
2 cloves garlic, minced
2 teaspoons Worcestershire sauce
1 teaspoon sugar
$1/4$ teaspoon basil
$1/8$ teaspoon oregano
$1/2$ cup Italian seasoned bread crumbs
$1/3$ cup Parmesan cheese
$1/2$ tablespoon margarine
2 ounces part-skim mozzarella

Cut tofu cake in half, and drain in colander one-half to 1 hour. Cut into strips about 1" x 3".

In a large saucepan, combine tomato sauce, garlic, Worcestershire sauce, sugar, basil, and oregano. Simmer on moderate heat 5 minutes. Let cool. Add tofu strips and marinate 30 minutes.

Preheat oven to 350 degrees. Grease a shallow baking pan with the margarine. Combine bread crumbs and Parmesan cheese. Remove tofu from sauce and dredge in crumb mixture. Place in pan in a single layer. Bake 15 minutes, turning strips once to brown evenly.

Cover with tomato sauce and sprinkle with mozzarella cheese. Return to oven for 5-10 minutes, until cheese is bubbly.

Serves 4.

Calcium per serving: 34% U.S. RDA
Calories per serving: 240

Note: Calcium content is based on tofu coagulated with calcium sulfate or calcium chloride.

Tofu Oriental Rice

16 ounces tofu (made with calcium sulfate or calcium chloride)
1 can (8 oz) unsweetened pineapple tidbits
2 cloves garlic, minced
$^1/_4$ cup light soy sauce
1" slice fresh ginger root, finely sliced (about 1 Tbsp)
1 tablespoon sherry wine
$^3/_4$ cup brown rice, uncooked
1 tablespoon oil
$^1/_2$ cup chopped green onions
$^1/_2$ cup chopped celery
2 cups bok choy, 1-inch slices
$^1/_2$ cup chopped green pepper
$^1/_2$ pound broccoli stems (sliced) and flowerets

Cut tofu cake in half, and drain in colander for one-half to 1 hour. Cut into $^3/_4$-inch cubes.

Combine 1/3 cup pineapple juice (drained from can), garlic, soy sauce, ginger, and sherry. Marinate tofu in mixture for several hours; drain, reserving marinade.

Cook rice according to package directions.

Heat oil in frying pan. Slowly brown tofu on all sides, handling gently to prevent crumbling. Remove from pan. In same pan combine onions, celery, bok choy, green pepper, broccoli, and reserved marinade. Cover and simmer about 5 minutes. Add pineapple tidbits with remaining juice, tofu, and cooked rice, and simmer a few minutes.

Serves 6.

Calcium per serving: 18% U.S. RDA
Calories per serving: 224

Note: calcium content is based on tofu coagulated with calcium sulfate or calcium chloride.

Sardine Muffin Pizza

1 English muffin, split
1 can (3 $^3/_4$ oz) sardines (with skin and bones)
2 tablespoons chopped red onions
$^1/_2$ cup tomato sauce
$^1/_8$ teaspoon basil
$^1/_8$ teaspoon oregano
$^1/_2$ garlic clove, minced
$^1/_2$ teaspoon sugar
2 tablespoons grated part-skim mozzarella
1 tablespoon grated Parmesan cheese

Preheat oven to 350 degrees. Toast the English muffin.

Drain the sardines and place on muffin halves. Sprinkle with chopped onions.

Combine tomato sauce, basil, oregano, garlic, and sugar in a small pan and cook over low heat 5 minutes. Pour over muffins, and sprinkle with mozzarella and Parmesan cheese. Bake until cheese melts, about 5 minutes.

Serves 2.

Calcium per serving: 35% U.S. RDA
Calories per serving: 234

Note: A Thomas brand plain English muffin contains more calcium than the same brand of honey wheat English muffin.

Sauces

For a thinner sauce for cream soups, reduce margarine and flour to 1 Tbsp each.

Cream Sauce No. 1, made with fluid milk

1 cup skim milk
2 tablespoons margarine
2 tablespoons flour
$^1/_8$ teaspoon salt, or to taste

Heat milk to almost boiling. Melt the margarine in a saucepan on moderate heat until it starts to bubble. Gradually stir in flour and salt with a wire whisk until well blended; do not allow to brown. Add hot milk, stirring vigorously with a wire whisk, and continue stirring until mixture comes to a boil and thickens. Lower heat and simmer 5 minutes or until desired consistency is reached. Makes about 1 cup.

Calcium ($^1/_4$ cup): 8% U.S. RDA
Calories ($^1/_4$ cup): 92

Cream Sauce No. 2, made with instant nonfat dry milk

$^1/_2$ cup instant nonfat dry milk
1 cup water (or canned chicken broth)
2 tablespoons margarine
2 tablespoons flour
$^1/_8$ teaspoon salt, or to taste (omit if using canned broth)
Pepper to taste

Mix dry milk with water and heat to almost boiling. Set aside.

Melt the margarine in a saucepan on moderate heat; gradually stir in flour with a wire whisk until well blended, but do not allow to brown. Add hot milk, stirring constantly with wire whisk until mixture comes to a boil and thickens. Lower heat and simmer 5 minutes or until desired consistency is reached. Makes about 1 cup.

Calcium ($^1/_4$ cup): 10% U.S. RDA
Calories ($^1/_4$ cup): 94

Cream Sauce No. 3, made with evaporated skimmed milk

$^2/_3$ cup canned evaporated skimmed milk, undiluted (divided)
2 tablespoons flour
$^1/_8$ teaspoon salt (omit if using canned broth)
Pepper to taste
$^1/_3$ cup water (or canned chicken broth)

Combine $^1/_4$ cup milk, flour, salt and pepper in small saucepan, and stir with a wire whisk until well blended. Add water and remaining milk, and cook on moderate heat, stirring constantly, until mixture thickens and comes to a boil. Makes about 1 cup.

Calcium ($^1/_4$ cup): 12% U.S. RDA
Calories ($^1/_4$ cup): 47

Cheese Sauce

1 recipe Cream Sauce
$^1/_4$ cup grated Parmesan or Romano cheese (or $^1/_2$ cup grated Cheddar, Colby, Gruyere, or Swiss)
$^1/_4$ teaspoon dry mustard, optional

Follow directions for selected cream sauce. After sauce begins to thicken, add grated cheese and stir with wire whisk on low heat just until cheese melts. Dry mustard may be added to sharpen the flavor.

Calcium and calorie content will vary, depending on which cheese and cream sauce is used.

Vegetables

A few words about greens

Greens are all good sources of calcium. By greens, we are referring to the group of vegetables that includes beet greens, collard greens, dandelion greens, kale, mustard greens, Swiss chard, and turnip greens. The flavors of the different greens vary from mild, somewhat like spinach (Swiss chard) to sharply pungent (mustard greens).

Greens can be prepared in an endless variety of tasty ways. Cooked for hours and served with cornbread, they have been a staple of Southerners for generations. Most recipes for spinach can be adapted for any type of greens. In recipes specifying a particular green, you can always substitute another one, or combine two or more greens. Once you've sampled various greens, you'll recognize their versatility for soups, stir-fry dishes, and vegetable casseroles. If you pick greens fresh from the garden, the young tender leaves of kale, Swiss chard, and dandelion greens may be added raw to lettuce salads.

How to cook greens

A traditional cooking method is to pile a variety of fresh pungent greens into a large pot of water together with a ham hock or chunks of salt pork, and then simmer for several hours. When the greens are eaten, the "pot liquor" (the broth remaining in the pot) is soaked up with pieces of cornbread.

The freshness, and thus the tenderness, of the vegetable determines the cooking time; freshly-picked, tender greens require less trimming, and need only be simmered for a short time in a small amount of water. Another method of cooking most greens (except collards) is to saute in a small amount of olive oil or cooking oil and then cover for 5-10 minutes until tender. However, the oil adds calories and fat.

The cooking time given for each green is approximate. The best test for tenderness is to taste a leaf at the end of the suggested cooking time, and cook longer if it is not tender enough for your taste. If you're in a hurry, shred the greens into smaller pieces, either by cutting them with a knife or putting them into a food processor for a few seconds.

It is important to wash fresh greens thoroughly, keeping in mind that the curlier the leaf, the more times it will need to be rinsed. Wash by dunking in a sink filled with cold water, then lifting out carefully so that any sand or debris stays in the sink. Drain, and repeat until water stays clear.

Add a tablespoon or two of lemon juice or vinegar to the cooking water of all greens to reduce the oxalic acid content and improve the flavor.

Cheezy Chard

1 pound fresh Swiss chard
2 tablespoons lemon juice
6 ounces plain nonfat yogurt
2 tablespoons grated Parmesan cheese
1 clove garlic, minced
1 teaspoon chopped chives

Wash chard thoroughly and discard stems. Cut leaves from midribs. Cook midribs in $^3/_4$ cup boiling salted water about 15 minutes. Add leaves and lemon juice and cook 10 minutes longer. (If the chard is young and tender, the leaves and midribs may be cooked together for 10-15 minutes.) Drain; chop coarsely.

Combine yogurt, cheese, garlic, and chives in a saucepan; add chard and heat mixture on low heat. Do not bring to a boil. Serves 4.

Calcium per serving: 18% U.S. RDA
Calories per serving: 57

Creole Okra

$^3/_4$ pound fresh okra pods, crowns removed, cut into $1^1/_2$-inch pieces
$^1/_2$ tablespoon oil
$^1/_2$ cup *each* chopped onions, celery, and green pepper
2 medium tomatoes, quartered
$^1/_2$ cup tomato juice
2 garlic cloves, minced
6 ounces plain nonfat yogurt
1 teaspoon Dijon-style mustard

Heat oil in frying pan, add onions and cook until transparent. Add okra and cook 5 minutes, turning over gently with spatula to cook evenly. Add celery, green pepper, tomatoes, tomato juice, and garlic and cook 5 minutes, stirring occasionally.

Combine yogurt and mustard. Add to vegetables and heat slowly to desired temperature. Do not bring to a boil. Serves 6.

Calcium per serving: 10% U.S. RDA
Calories per serving: 61

Crunchy Kale

1^1/$_2$ pounds fresh kale
4 tablespoons lemon juice (divided)
^{3}/$_4$ cup sliced onions
^{1}/$_2$ tablespoon margarine
1 clove garlic, minced
^{1}/$_2$ cup red bell pepper, chopped
1 tablespoon sesame seeds

Wash kale thoroughly and discard stems. Cut into 2-inch strips. Add 2 tablespoons lemon juice to ^{1}/$_2$ cup water; bring to a boil and add kale. Simmer, covered, for about 10-15 minutes. Drain.

In another pan, saute onions in margarine until lightly browned. Add 2 tablespoons lemon juice and garlic, stirring to blend. Add kale and chopped red pepper, and cook on low heat 5 minutes.

Heat small frying pan on moderate heat until drop of water sizzles. Add sesame seeds and stir continuously until lightly browned. Sprinkle seeds over each serving.

Serves 4.

Calcium per serving: 12% U.S. RDA
Calories per serving: 69

Glazed Beets and Greens

2 pounds beet greens
2 tablespoons lemon juice
4 beets
1 tablespoon cornstarch
$^1/_2$ cup orange juice
1 tablespoon brown sugar

Cut greens from beets and wash thoroughly. Cut into 2-inch strips. Add lemon juice to $^1/_2$ cup salted water and bring to a boil. Add greens to pan, cover, and simmer about 8 minutes. Drain.

Wash beets thoroughly; cut off all but 1 inch of stems and discard. Cook beets in 1 cup salted water 30-45 minutes, until tender. Drain, reserving 1/3 cup liquid. Peel beets, and when cool, cut into strips.

Make a paste of cornstarch and reserved beet liquid. Combine with orange juice and brown sugar in a medium saucepan. Cook over moderate heat until mixture comes to a boil. Lower heat, add beets and greens, and simmer 5 minutes. Serves 4.

Calcium per serving: 9% U.S. RDA
Calories per serving: 65

Spicy Turnip Greens

$1^1/_4$ pounds fresh turnip greens
2 tablespoons lemon juice
$^1/_2$ cup apple juice
1 medium apple, grated
1-inch slice fresh ginger, finely sliced (or $^1/_4$ tsp ground)
$^1/_2$ teaspoon coriander
$^1/_2$ cup plain nonfat yogurt

Wash turnip greens thoroughly. Add lemon juice to $^3/_4$ cup salted water and bring to a boil. Add greens and cook, covered, 20-25 minutes. Remove from pan and drain. In same pan, combine apple juice, apple, ginger, and coriander; add greens and cook on moderate heat 5 minutes. Stir in yogurt and warm on low heat. Do not boil. Serves 4.

Calcium per serving: 16% U.S. RDA
Calories per serving: 75

Georgia Collards

1¼ pounds fresh collard greens
2 tablespoons lemon juice
½ cup chopped onions
½ tablespoon margarine
½ tablespoon flour
⅔ cup apple juice
2 tablespoons cider vinegar
2 tablespoons sugar
¼ teaspoon dry mustard

Wash collards thoroughly and discard stems. Slice into 2-inch strips. Add lemon juice to ½ cup salted water; bring to a boil and add collards. Simmer, covered, about 20 minutes. Drain.

Saute onions in margarine until lightly browned. Stir in flour with wire whisk; add apple juice, vinegar, sugar, and mustard. Cook over moderate heat, stirring constantly, until mixture thickens. Add collards to sauce and cook 5 minutes on low heat, stirring frequently.

Serves 4.

Calcium per serving: 12% U.S. RDA
Calories per serving: 90

Mustard Greens Oriental

1^{1}/$_{4}$ pound fresh mustard greens
2 tablespoons lemon juice
^{1}/$_{2}$ chicken bouillon cube
^{1}/$_{2}$ cup water
^{1}/$_{2}$ cup chopped green onions
2 tablespoons light soy sauce
1 clove garlic, minced
8 ounces raw mushrooms, sliced
^{1}/$_{2}$ cup mung bean sprouts
^{1}/$_{3}$ cup sliced water chestnuts

Wash mustard greens very thoroughly until rinse water is clear. Cut into 2-inch strips.

Add lemon juice to ^{1}/$_{2}$ cup water, and bring to a boil. Add greens and cook, covered, about 15 minutes. Drain.

Heat ^{1}/$_{2}$ cup water to boiling and add bouillon cube, stirring to dissolve. Add onions, soy sauce, and garlic, and simmer 3-4 minutes. Mix in greens, mushrooms, bean sprouts, and water chestnuts. Cover pan and cook until sprouts are wilted.

Serves 4.

Calcium per serving: 12% U.S. RDA
Calories per serving: 90

Desserts

Grammy's Rum-Raisin Rice Pudding

1$\frac{1}{2}$ cups evaporated skimmed milk, undiluted (divided)
$\frac{1}{2}$ cup water
Salt to taste
$\frac{1}{4}$ cup uncooked white rice
$\frac{1}{3}$ cup raisins
1 tablespoon water
2 eggs
2 tablespoons brown sugar
1 tablespoon granulated sugar
1 cup skim milk
1 tablespoon rum (or 1 tsp rum extract)
Sprinkle of nutmeg

Preheat oven to 350 degrees. In a saucepan, combine $\frac{1}{2}$ cup evaporated skimmed milk, $\frac{1}{2}$ cup water, and a pinch of salt. Bring to a bubbling simmer on moderate heat. Add rice gradually and return to a simmer. Cover and lower heat; cook until rice absorbs all of the liquid, about 20 minutes.

Combine raisins and 1 tablespoon water in small pan. Heat until water just starts to boil, then cover pan and remove from heat.

Beat eggs with brown sugar, granulated sugar, and a pinch of salt.

Combine 1 cup evaporated skimmed milk and 1 cup skim milk and heat until mixture scalds. Remove from heat and pour slowly into egg mixture, beating with a wire whisk. Mix in rice, raisins, and rum. Pour into a greased glass loaf pan and sprinkle with nutmeg.

Place loaf pan into a larger pan; add hot water to outer pan to a depth of 1 inch. Bake 30-35 minutes until top is lightly browned.

Serves 6.

Calcium per serving: 25% U.S. RDA
Calories per serving: 164

Cocoa Pudding

1 tablespoon cornstarch
2 $\frac{1}{2}$ cups plus 2 tablespoons fluid skim milk (divided)
$\frac{1}{4}$ cup unsweetened cocoa
$\frac{1}{3}$ cup nonfat instant dry milk
$\frac{1}{4}$ cup sugar
1 egg
$\frac{1}{2}$ teaspoon vanilla

Mix cornstarch with 2 tablespoons fluid milk to make a smooth paste.

In a saucepan, combine cocoa, dry milk, and sugar. Add egg, $\frac{1}{2}$ cup fluid milk, and cornstarch paste. Stir vigorously with a wire whisk. Place pan on moderate heat; add remaining fluid milk and cook until mixture just comes to a boil, stirring frequently with a wire whisk. Lower heat and simmer 3-4 minutes, stirring constantly.

Remove pan from heat and stir in vanilla. Pour into 5 custard cups. Refrigerate.

Serves 5.

Calcium per serving: 22% U.S. RDA
Calories per serving: 130

Blueberry Pudding Parfait

1 package (3 ½ oz) vanilla pudding (not instant), made with
2 cups skim milk
1½ cups fresh blueberries
Yogurt cream cheese (made from 16 oz vanilla-flavored yogurt,
    drained 3-4 hrs)

Prepare pudding according to package directions. Reserve ¼ cup blueberries.

Layer ingredients in 6 parfait glasses, as follows: half of the blueberries, divided among the glasses; 1 tablespoon of yogurt cream cheese in each glass; 1 cup of the pudding, divided among the glasses. Repeat with a second layer, then sprinkle with reserved berries.

Serves 6.

Calcium per serving: 14% U.S. RDA
Calories per serving: 169

Variations:

For a Fourth of July treat, alternate layers of sliced strawberries with the blueberries.

Layer chocolate pudding with vanilla-flavored yogurt cream cheese (drained 3-4 hrs), and sprinkle chopped nuts between layers.

Layer lemon pudding with lemon-flavored yogurt cream cheese (drained 3-4 hrs), and sprinkle flaked coconut between layers.

Pina Colada Sorbet

$1/3$ cup sugar
1 envelope unflavored gelatin
$1/2$ cup unsweetened crushed pineapple
2 cups buttermilk
1 teaspoon coconut extract
1 teaspoon rum extract
1 egg white

Combine sugar, gelatin, and $1/4$ cup pineapple juice (drained from can) in a saucepan, and place on very low heat. Stir until gelatin is completely dissolved. Cool.

Combine buttermilk, coconut extract, and rum extract in a bowl. Add gelatin mixture and mix well with a wire whisk. Pour into a glass loaf pan and place in freezer until ice forms a 2-inch rim around the edge (about $1^1/2$-2 hrs). Place a mixing bowl in freezer to chill.

Spoon mixture into the chilled bowl. Add egg white and pineapple, and beat with electric mixer for about 5 minutes on highest speed. Return mixture to pan (which has been rinsed in cold water), and return to freezer for several hours.

Serve with fresh strawberries, if desired. For a creamier texture, remove from freezer, beat 5 minutes, and refreeze before serving.

Serves 6.

Calcium per serving: 10% U.S. RDA
Calories per serving: 100

Yogurt Cream Cheese Cake

4 graham crackers (2 $1/2$-inch squares)
$1/2$ tablespoon margarine
Yogurt cream cheese (made from 16 oz low fat lemon yogurt,
    drained 12-14 hrs)
Yogurt cream cheese (made from 16 oz low fat vanilla yogurt,
    drained 12-14 hrs)
$3/4$ cup evaporated skimmed milk
1 tablespoon lemon juice
$1/4$ cup sugar
1 teaspoon grated lemon peel
3 eggs, separated
1 egg white

Frosting (optional)
Yogurt cream cheese (made from 8 oz vanilla yogurt, drained 3-4 hrs)

Preheat oven to 350 degrees.

Crush graham crackers with rolling pin (or use blender or food processor). Spread bottom and sides of an 8" pie plate with margarine, then sprinkle with crumbs, rotating plate to spread evenly.

Combine vanilla yogurt cream cheese, lemon yogurt cream cheese, evaporated milk, lemon juice, sugar, grated lemon peel, and egg yolks; blend well.

Beat egg whites until stiff peaks form. Gently fold in yogurt cream cheese mixture with rubber spatula. Spread evenly over crumbs in pie plate.

Bake 40 minutes, until very lightly browned. Leave in oven with door ajar about 15 minutes, then remove from oven and let cool at room temperature. Refrigerate several hours before serving.

Spread with yogurt cream cheese, if desired, and serve with fresh strawberries on top.

Serves 8.

Calcium per serving: 19% U.S. RDA (22% with frosting)
Calories per serving: 150 (164 with frosting)

Rhuberry Mousse

$^2/_3$ cup evaporated skimmed milk, undiluted
1 pound fresh rhubarb, diced (or unsweetened frozen)
$^1/_3$ cup sugar
$^3/_4$ cup orange juice (divided)
2 envelopes unsweetened gelatin
16 ounces sweetened frozen sliced strawberries (thawed)

Place can of evaporated milk in refrigerator 12 hours, or freeze for 30 minutes. Chill a 2-quart bowl in the freezer for 15 minutes.

Combine rhubarb, sugar, and $^1/_2$ cup orange juice in a saucepan. Cover and cook over moderate heat, stirring occasionally, until rhubarb is tender, about 15 minutes.

In another saucepan, combine gelatin and $^1/_4$ cup orange juice and stir over very low heat until gelatin dissolves. Add to rhubarb. Mix in strawberries. Pour into loaf pan and refrigerate for about 30-45 minutes, until mixture thickens and starts to set.

Pour cold evaporated milk into cold bowl and whip on high speed until soft peaks are formed. Fold in rhubarb mixture. Pour into serving dish and refrigerate at least 4 hours or overnight.

Serve with sliced fresh strawberries on top.

Serves 6.

Calcium per serving: 16% U.S. RDA
Calories per serving: 173

Maple-Fig Tapioca Pudding

3 Calimyrna figs, chopped
2 cups skim milk
1 egg, separated
3 tablespoons granulated quick-cooking tapioca
2 tablespoons brown sugar
1 tablespoon sugar
$1/4$ teaspoon maple flavoring

Cook figs in 2 tablespoons water over moderate heat; stir constantly until water evaporates, about 1-2 minutes. Remove from heat.

In a saucepan, mix milk and egg yolk with a wire whisk. Add tapioca and brown sugar. Cook over moderate heat, stirring constantly until mixture comes to a boil. Stir in maple flavoring and remove from heat.

Beat egg white in a medium bowl, gradually adding sugar until soft peaks form. Slowly pour tapioca mixture into beaten egg white, stirring with wire whisk until completely blended.

Spoon figs into 4 custard cups and pour in tapioca mixture. Refrigerate.

Serves 4.

Calcium per serving: 18% U.S. RDA
Calories per serving: 158

Whipped Cream No. 1, made with evaporated skimmed milk

$^1/_2$ cup canned evaporated skimmed milk
1 tablespoon lemon juice
2 tablespoons confectioners' sugar

Prepare within 1 hour of serving. Chill milk in refrigerator for about 8 hours, or about 45 minutes in the freezer. Chill mixing bowl and beaters in freezer for about 15 minutes.

Beat milk with electric mixer on highest speed until soft peaks start to form. Add lemon juice and sugar, and continue beating until mixture forms stiff peaks. Refrigerate. Makes about 3 cups (volume is variable).

Calcium (1 cup): about 12% U.S. RDA
Calories (1 cup): about 49

Whipped Cream No. 2, made with instant nonfat dry milk

$^1/_2$ cup instant nonfat dry milk
$^1/_3$ cup cold water (or cold fruit juice)
2 teaspoons lemon juice
$1^1/_2$ tablespoons confectioners' sugar

Prepare within 1 hour of serving. Chill small mixing bowl and beaters in freezer about 15 minutes.

Beat milk and water with electric mixer at highest speed until soft peaks start to form. Add lemon juice and sugar, and continue beating until stiff peaks form. Refrigerate. Makes about 3 cups (volume is variable).

Calcium (1 cup): about 14% U.S. RDA
Calories (1 cup): about 53 (if made with water)

Calories added if made with fruit juice: apple juice 13, apricot nectar 16, cranberry juice 18, orange juice 13, pineapple juice 16

For comparison, 1 cup of regular whipped cream, from $^1/_2$ cup of whipping cream, has 410 calories and 8% of the U.S. RDA for calcium.

Kiddie Calcium

If coaxing, gentle persuasion, or even bribery has failed to convince your children to drink more milk, there are other ways they can get the calcium their growing bones need — from cheese, yogurt, yogurt cream cheese, from dairy products "hidden" in foods they like, and from high calcium recipes.

Most children who shove away a glass of milk will reach eagerly for a sweet pudding or other high calcium dessert and never suspect they're getting all the nutritional benefits of milk. Even those who turn up their noses at a grilled cheese sandwich are fascinated by "strip" or "string" cheese, which is fun to eat.

Most of the ideas and recipes that follow will appeal to young children and teens, as well as to adults.

Flavor Your Own Yogurt

Kids who say they don't like yogurt probably haven't tasted all the new types and flavors, and there should be several to satisfy even the most finicky eater. Even better than store-bought may be yogurt combinations created by the kids themselves. Let them experiment by mixing a small carton of plain yogurt with some fresh fruit and/or a teaspoon of brown sugar, honey, maple syrup, or jam, or a tablespoon or more of peanut butter or their favorite breakfast cereal.

Cheese Snacks, Cheese Balls

Kids who won't eat properly are more likely to snack properly, with your guidance. Children who like to help in the kitchen can mix yogurt cream cheese with their favorite flavoring ingredients. They can snack on their creation spread on graham crackers, celery sticks, carrot sticks, or banana slices. Or they can form the mixture into balls, which can be eaten plain or rolled in breakfast cereal crumbs. Refrigerate the balls after mixing and handling, to allow them to firm up.

Yogurt cream cheese balls made with vanilla- or lemon-flavored yogurt can be sandwiched between two graham crackers or wafer cookies for a sweet treat.

162

Cheese Popcorn

Kids of all ages (and their parents) find it hard to resist the aroma of freshly popped corn. Popcorn, by itself, contains no calcium, but you can add some cheese for a calcium-boosting snack.

Put the freshly-popped popcorn into a baking pan and sprinkle with their favorite cheese, grated. Mix together with a fork, and heat in a 300 degree oven until the cheese is melted, about 5-8 minutes.

Cheese Muffins

1³/₄ cups flour
1 tablespoon baking powder
1 tablespoon sugar
³/₄ cup grated Swiss cheese
1 egg
1 cup buttermilk
3 tablespoons margarine, melted and cooled

Preheat oven to 375 degrees. Sift together flour, baking powder, and sugar. Stir grated cheese into dry ingredients with a fork.

Beat egg, milk, and melted margarine with a wire whisk until well blended. Add dry ingredients to milk mixture, stirring just until batter is evenly moistened.

Spoon into 12 greased muffin tins and bake 25-30 minutes, until tops are lightly browned. Serve immediately. (May be reheated in a 350 degree oven for about 5 minutes.)

Makes 12 muffins.

Calcium per muffin: 11% U.S. RDA
Calories per muffin: 131

The Yogurt Cheezapple

An ordinary apple is not ordinarily a good source of calcium. Nor is it what most children would consider their ideal snack. Yet an apple is a good snack because it's filling, it's an excellent source of natural fiber (especially if you don't peel it), and it contains vitamin C and other valuable nutrients. The challenge is to give your children all these nutritional "goodies" plus calcium, *and* make it appealing to them. How?

The answer is the Yogurt Cheezapple! The recipe is simple: 1 Delicious apple plus any yogurt cream cheese spread (recipes follow).

Core the apple, cutting out the seeds. Cut into 8 wedges-shaped sections. Keeping the sections in their original order (place in a small bowl), remove a section and spread one side with the selected spread. Return to its original position and repeat with the next section. Continue until there is yogurt cream cheese filling between all the sections.

Fill the center with any remaining filling. Wipe the outside of the apple with a dampened paper towel to remove any smeared filling. Refrigerate for several hours.

Apple-Honey Spread

Yogurt cream cheese (made from 8 oz plain low fat yogurt,
    drained 12-14 hrs)
1 tablespoon frozen apple juice concentrate
1 tablespoon corn flake crumbs
1 teaspoon honey

Combine all ingredients. Refrigerate several hours. Makes about $1/2$ cup.

Calcium (1 oz): 6% U.S.RDA
Calories (1 oz): 66

Citrus-Cinnamon Spread

Yogurt cream cheese (made from 8 oz lemon-flavored yogurt,
    drained 12-14 hrs)
1 teaspoon orange marmalade
$1/2$ teaspoon grated lemon peel
$1/2$ teaspoon grated orange peel

Combine all ingredients. Refrigerate several hours. Makes about $1/2$ cup.

Calcium (1 oz): 6% U.S. RDA
Calories (1 oz): 51

Peanut-Raisin Spread

1 tablespoon raisins
Yogurt cream cheese (made from 8 oz plain nonfat yogurt,
    drained 12-14 hrs)
1 tablespoon peanut butter

Combine all ingredients. Refrigerate several hours. Makes about $1/2$ cup.

Calcium (1 oz): 7% U.S. RDA
Calories (1 oz): 61

Peanut Butter and Jellysicle

$3/4$ cup grape juice
2 tablespoons grape jam or jelly
1 envelope unflavored gelatin
16 ounces plain low fat yogurt
$1/4$ cup creamy peanut butter
$1/2$ cup skim milk
8 paper or plastic cups (3 oz size)
8 wooden sticks (called building sticks at hobby & toy stores)

In a small pan, combine grape juice, grape jam, and gelatin. Stir over low heat until gelatin is dissolved. Remove from heat, and let cool for a few minutes.

With a wire whisk, blend yogurt, peanut butter, and milk. Add cooled gelatin mixture and blend thoroughly. Pour into glass loaf pan and place in freezer. When ice crystals have formed a 2-inch rim around the edge of pan (about $1^1/2$-2 hrs), place a medium mixing bowl and beaters in freezer for about 15 minutes.

Remove pan from freezer, and spoon mixture into chilled bowl; beat with electric mixer at high speed for 3-5 minutes. Spoon into cups and return to freezer. After about 30 minutes, insert sticks.

Remove from freezer a few minutes before serving. Remove cups.

Makes 8.

Calcium per serving: 12% U.S. RDA
Calories per serving: 130

Pineapple-Banana Pop

3 tablespoons frozen pineapple juice concentrate (thawed)
2 tablespoons honey
3 tablespoons water
1 envelope unflavored gelatin
2 ripe bananas, mashed (1 cup)
16 ounces low fat vanilla-flavored yogurt
$1/3$ cup evaporated skimmed milk
10 paper or plastic cups (3 oz size)
10 wooden sticks (called building sticks at hobby and toy stores)

In a small pan, combine frozen concentrate, honey, water, and gelatin; stir over low heat until gelatin is dissolved. Remove from heat and let cool for a few minutes.

Mix mashed bananas and yogurt with a wire whisk; add evaporated milk and gelatin mixture and blend thoroughly. Pour into a glass loaf pan and place in freezer. When ice crystals have formed a 2-inch rim around the edge of the pan (about $1^1/2$-2 hrs), place a medium mixing bowl in freezer, together with beaters, for about 15 minutes.

Remove pan from freezer and spoon mixture into the chilled bowl; beat with electric mixer at high speed for about 3-5 minutes. Spoon into cups and return to freezer. After about 30 minutes, insert sticks.

Remove from freezer a few minutes before serving. Remove cups.

Makes 10.

Calcium per serving: 10% U.S. RDA
Calories per serving: 88

Cran-Strawberry Pop

1 envelope unflavored gelatin
2 tablespoons sugar
3 tablespoons cranberry juice
1 tablespoon water
1 cup crushed fresh strawberries (about 1 pint)
16 ounces plain low fat yogurt
8 paper or plastic cups (3 oz size)
8 wooden sticks (called building sticks at hobby and toy stores)

In a small saucepan, combine gelatin, sugar, cranberry juice, and water. Stir over low heat until gelatin is dissolved. Remove from heat and let cool for a few minutes.

Crush strawberries in a food processor or blender. Stir in yogurt, then add cooled gelatin mixture. Whisk vigorously with a wire whisk. Pour into a glass loaf pan and place in freezer. When ice crystals have formed a 2-inch rim around edge of pan (about $1^1/2$-2 hrs), place a medium bowl and beaters in freezer for 15 minutes.

Remove pan from freezer and beat with electric mixer for about 5 minutes. Spoon into cups and return to freezer. Insert sticks after about 30 minutes. Remove from freezer a few minutes before serving. Remove cups. Makes 8.

Calcium per serving: 10% U.S. RDA
Calories per serving: 69

Apple Shake

$3/4$ cup skim milk
1 tablespoon frozen apple juice concentrate (thawed)
$1/4$ cup canned unsweetened applesauce
1 tablespoon instant nonfat dry milk
Sprinkle of cinnamon

Mix all ingredients in a blender or food processor until smooth. Serves 1.

Calcium: 28% U.S. RDA
Calories: 128

Apricot Shake

$^3/_4$ cup buttermilk
$^1/_4$ cup apricot nectar
1 tablespoon instant nonfat dry milk
Sprinkle of coriander

Mix all ingredients in a blender or food processor until smooth. Serves 1.

Calcium: 27% U.S. RDA
Calories: 122

Banana Colada Shake

$^3/_4$ cup skim milk
$^1/_2$ banana, mashed
1 tablespoon instant nonfat dry milk
$^1/_4$ teaspoon coconut extract

Mix all ingredients in a blender or food processor until smooth. Serves 1.

Calcium: 28% U.S. RDA
Calories: 131

Peach Shake

$^3/_4$ cup skim milk
$^1/_4$ cup fresh sliced peaches, peeled
1 tablespoon instant nonfat dry milk
Sprinkle of nutmeg

Mix all ingredients in a blender or food processor until smooth. Serves 1.

Calcium: 28% U.S. RDA
Calories: 107

PART IV

CALCIUM AND CALORIE COUNTER

11

CALCIUM AND CALORIE COUNTER FOR THE SUPERMARKET

THIS SHOPPING guide provides the calcium and calorie contents of a broad variety of fresh and brand name foods, so you can quickly and easily determine which are the best bone-builders. For your convenience when shopping, the foods are grouped by departments of the supermarket (in alphabetical order):

> Dairy (includes non-dairy refrigerated foods)
> Fresh fish
> Frozen foods
> Grocery (canned and packaged foods)
> Produce

The calcium in each food is given as a percentage of the U.S. RDA. You can easily compare similar products to determine which ones contain the most calcium and fewest calories.

The indicated serving size should be noted when making calorie and calcium comparisons. For example, a yogurt carton may contain 6 or 8 ounces; the indicated serving sizes of frozen lasagna range from 9 $1/2$ to 11 ounces.

To determine your own daily calcium intake, just add up the percentages of each food you consume. You may be surprised to discover how quickly the percentages mount up, especially when your diet has a dairy base of milk, yogurt and/or cheese.

Since only a very limited number of food products could be included in this shopping guide, the omission of any food does not mean that it is not a good source of calcium. You should check the nutrition information label of any brand name foods that you rely on regularly as a calcium source, since the nutritional contents may change periodically.

171

The nutritional information (and serving size) for each brand name food was provided by the food manufacturer. Data on fresh foods was obtained from the latest nutritional information issued by the U.S. Department of Agriculture.

Dairy Products
(Including non-dairy refrigerated foods)

Cheese, Cottage (see Cottage Cheese)

Cheese, Natural

FOOD / BRAND NAME	SERVING	CALORIES	CALCIUM % U.S. RDA
Blue			
Kraft	1 oz	100	15%
Sargento	1 oz	100	15%
Brie (Sargento)	1 oz	95	6%
Brick			
Kraft	1 oz	110	20%
Sargento	1 oz	110	20%
Camembert			
Kraft	1 oz	90	12%
Sargento	1 oz	90	12%
Caraway (Kraft)	1 oz	100	15%
Cheddar			
Kraft, mild or sharp	1 oz	110	20%
Kraft, Cracker Barrel	1 oz	110	20%
Colby			
Kraft	1 oz	110	20%
Land O Lakes	1 oz	110	20%
Sargento	1 oz	110	20%
Edam			
Kraft	1 oz	90	20%
Land O Lakes	1 oz	100	20%
Farmers (Sargento)	1 oz	100	20%
Fetz (Sargento)	1 oz	80	14%
Fontina (Sargento)	1 oz	110	16%

Cheese, natural *(continued)*

FOOD / BRAND NAME	SERVING	CALORIES	CALCIUM % U.S. RDA
Gjetost (Sargento)	1 oz	130	11%
Gouda			
Kraft	1 oz	110	15%
Land O Lakes	1 oz	100	20%
Gruyere (Sargento)	1 oz	120	30%
Limburger			
Mohawk Valley (Little Gem)	1 oz	100	15%
Monterey jack			
Kraft	1 oz	110	20%
Land O Lakes	1 oz	110	20%
Mozzarella, low moisture			
Kraft, part skim	1 oz	80	20%
Sargento, part skim	1 oz	80	20%
Sargento, whole milk	1 oz	90	15%
Muenster			
Kraft Casino	1 oz	110	20%
Sargento	1 oz	100	20%
Neufchatel (Kraft)	1 oz	80	2%
Parmesan			
Kraft	1 oz	110	30%
Kraft, grated	1 oz	130	40%
Sargento, grated	1 oz	130	40%
Provolone (Kraft, Sargento)	1 oz	100	20%
Ricotta			
Sargento, part skim	1 oz	30	6%
Sargento, whole milk	1 oz	50	8%
Romano			
Kraft, grated	1 oz	130	35%
Sargento	1 oz	110	30%
Scamorze, low moisture			
Kraft, part-skim	1 oz	80	20%
Swiss			
Kraft, aged chunk	1 oz	110	30%
Sargento, Finland	1 oz	110	30%
String (Sargento)	1 oz	80	20%

Pasteurized process cheese, cheese food, cheese spread and cheese product

FOOD / BRAND NAME	SERVING	CALORIES	CALCIUM % U.S. RDA
Pasteurized process cheese, cheese food, cheese spread and cheese product			
American			
bacon, with (Kraft)	1 oz	90	15%
bacon, with (Squeez-a-Snak)	1 oz	90	15%
Borden Lite-Line, singles	1 oz	50	20%
Borden cheese food, singles	1 oz	90	15%
Borden, Light American, singles	1 oz	70	20%
Golden Image	1 oz	90	20%
Harvest Moon	1 oz	70	20%
Kraft, grated	1 oz	70	15%
Kraft, singles	1 oz	90	15%
Kraft, spread	1 oz	80	15%
Kraft Deluxe, loaf	1 oz	110	20%
Kraft Deluxe, slices	1 oz	110	15%
Kraft Golden Image	1 oz	90	20%
LactAid lactose reduced	1 oz	90	10%
Land O Lakes	1 oz	110	15%
Light n' Lively, singles	1 oz	70	20%
Old English, sharp, loaf	1 oz	110	20%
Old English, sharp, slices	1 oz	110	15%
Swiss			
Land O Lakes	1 oz	100	20%
Weight Watchers	1 oz	50	20%
Blue, spread (Roka)	1 oz	70	6%
Caraway (Kraft)	1 oz	100	20%
Cheddar, singles (Light n' Lively)	1 oz	70	20%
Cheddar, sharp			
Borden Lite-Line	1 oz	50	20%
Cracker Barrel	1 oz	90	15%
Golden Image	1 oz	110	20%
Light n' Lively	1 oz	70	20%
Weight Watchers	1 oz	70	20%
Cheese wedges (Laughing Cow)	3/4 oz	54	8%
reduced calorie (Laughing Cow)	3/4 oz	35	10%
Cheez 'n bacon, singles (Kraft)	1 oz	100	15%

Cheese, processed *(continued)*

FOOD / BRAND NAME	SERVING	CALORIES	CALCIUM % U.S. RDA
Cheez Whiz spread	1 oz	80	10%
with jalapeno peppers	1 oz	80	15%
with pimento	1 oz	80	15%
Colby (Golden Image)	1 oz	110	20%
Cracker Barrel			
sharp cheddar cold pack	1 oz	90	15%
Garlic, with (Kraft)			
Golden Velvet cheese spread	1 oz	80	15%
Land O Lakes			
Harvest Moon, loaf	1 oz	50	10%
Jalapeno			
Kraft	1 oz	80	15%
Kraft, singles	1 oz	90	15%
Land O Lakes	1 oz	90	15%
LactAid, lactose reduced slices	1 oz	90	10%
Limburger, gem (Mohawk Valley)	1 oz	90	15%
Limburger spread (Mohawk Valley)	1 oz	70	10%
Low cholesterol singles (Borden Lite-Line)	1 oz	90	15%
Mexican Velveeta (Kraft)	1 oz	80	15%
Monterey jack (Kraft, singles)	1 oz	90	15%
w/caraway seeds (Casino)	1 oz	100	20%
w/jalapeno peppers (Casino)	1 oz	100	20%
Mozzarella, singles (Borden Lite-line)	1 oz	50	20%
Olives & pimento spread (Kraft)	1 oz	60	4%
Onion			
Land O Lakes	1 oz	90	20%
Weight Watchers	1 oz	70	20%
Pepperoni cheese food (Land O Lakes)	1 oz	90	15%
Pimento			
Kraft Deluxe	1 oz	110	15%
Kraft cheese spread	1 oz	80	15%
Kraft, singles	1 oz	90	15%
Kraft spread	1 oz	70	4%
Pineapple spread (Kraft)	1 oz	70	4%
Relish spread (Kraft)	1 oz	70	2%
Salami cheese food (Land O Lakes)	1 oz	100	15%

Cheese, processed *(continued)*

FOOD / BRAND NAME	SERVING	CALORIES	CALCIUM % U.S. RDA
Sharp cheddar			
Borden Lite-line	1 oz	50	20%
Cracker Barrel	1 oz	90	15%
Light n' Lively	1 oz	70	20%
Weight Watchers	1 oz	70	20%
Sharp process cheese spread			
Old English	1 oz	90	15%
Sharp, single slices			
Kraft	1 oz	100	15%
Old English	1 oz	110	15%
Single slices			
American			
Borden	1 oz	110	20%
Borden cheese food	1 oz	90	15%
Borden Lite-Line	1 oz	50	20%
Borden Light American	1 oz	70	10%
Kraft	1 oz	90	15%
Kraft Deluxe	1 oz	110	15%
Kraft Golden Image	1 oz	90	20%
Land O Lakes	3/4 oz	64	12%
Light n' Lively	1 oz	70	20%
Cheez 'n bacon (Kraft)	1 oz	100	15%
Jalapeno (Kraft)	1 oz	90	15%
Monterey jack (Kraft)	1 oz	90	15%
Mozzarella (Borden Lite-line)	1 oz	50	20%
Pimento			
Kraft	1 oz	90	15%
Kraft Deluxe	1 oz	100	15%
Sharp			
Kraft	1 oz	100	15%
Old English	1 oz	110	15%
Sharp cheddar			
Borden Lite-Line	1 oz	50	20%
Light n' Lively	1 oz	70	20%
Swiss			
Borden	1 oz	100	25%
Borden Lite-Line	1 oz	50	20%

Cheese, processed *(continued)*

FOOD / BRAND NAME	SERVING	CALORIES	CALCIUM % U.S. RDA
Kraft Deluxe	1 oz	90	20%
Kraft	1 oz	90	20%
Weight Watchers	1 oz	70	20%
Velveeta (Kraft)	1 oz	90	15%
Smoked cheese cold pack			
Weight Watchers	1 oz	70	20%
Smokelle	1 oz	100	20%
Squeez-a-Snak, w/bacon, garlic or pimento	1 oz	90	15%
Squeez-a-Snak, sharp or hickory-smoke	1 oz	80	15%
Swiss, single slices			
Borden	1 oz	100	25%
Kraft	1 oz	90	20%
Kraft Deluxe	1 oz	90	20%
Light 'n Lively	1 oz	70	20%
Taco (Sargento)	1 oz	110	20%
Taco, shredded (Kraft)	1 oz	110	20%
Velveeta, slices (Kraft)	1 oz	90	15%
Mexican, pimento, or spread	1 oz	80	15%
Wedges			
Laughing Cow	1 oz	70	15%
Laughing Cow, reduced calorie	³/₄ oz	35	12%

Cottage Cheese

Breakstone's			
dry curd	4 oz	90	15%
lowfat	4 oz	90	8%
smooth & creamy, tangy	4 oz	110	8%
w/pineapple	4 oz	140	6%
Light n' Lively	4 oz	80	10%
w/garden salad	4 oz	80	10%
w/peach & pineapple	4 oz	110	4%
Sealtest	4 oz	120	6%
w/garden salad	4 oz	120	6%
w/peach & pineapple	4 oz	140	4%

Cream

Half-and-half	1 Tbsp	20	*

Cream *(continued)*

FOOD / BRAND NAME	SERVING	CALORIES	CALCIUM % U.S. RDA
Light, coffee or table	1 Tbsp	30	*
Sour (*see* Sour Cream)			
Whipping (unwhipped)			
light	1 Tbsp	45	*
heavy	1 Tbsp	50	*

Cream cheese

Breakstone's, TempTee	1 oz	100	2%
Philadelphia			
light	1 oz	80	2%
regular or soft	1 oz	100	2%
soft w/chives & onion	1 oz	100	2%
soft w/pineapple or w/strawberries	1 oz	90	2%

Eggs

Egg	1	80	3%

Milk

Buttermilk	1 cup	100	28%
Chocolate			
1% fat (lowfat)	1 cup	160	29%
2% fat (lowfat)	1 cup	180	28%
whole	1 cup	210	28%
Lowfat			
1% (no added milk solids)	1 cup	100	30%
1% (milk solids added)	1 cup	105	31%
2% (no added milk solids)	1 cup	120	30%
2% (milk solids added)	1 cup	125	31%
Skim			
No added milk solids	1 cup	85	30%
Milk solids added	1 cup	90	31%
Whole (3.3% fat)	1 cup	150	29%

* Less than 2% U.S. RDA

Puddings, refrigerated

FOOD / BRAND NAME	SERVING	CALORIES	CALCIUM % U.S. RDA
Puddings, refrigerated			
Butterscotch (Swiss Miss)	4 oz	140	10%
Chocolate (Swiss Miss)	4 oz	150	10%
Chocolate fudge (Swiss Miss)	4 oz	170	10%
Chocolate w/fudge topping (Swiss Miss)	4 oz	170	8%
Tapioca (Swiss Miss)	4 oz	130	8%
Vanilla (Swiss Miss)	4 oz	140	10%
Vanilla w/fudge topping (Swiss Miss)	4 oz	160	6%
Sour Cream			
Breakstone's	1 oz	60	2%
Sealtest	1 oz	60	4%
Yogurt			
Amaretto almond (Yoplait YoCreme)	5 oz	240	35%
Apple, dutch apple			
Dannon	8 oz	240	35%
Yoplait original	6 oz	190	25%
Apple cinnamon (Yoplait breakfast)	6 oz	220	50%
Banana			
Dannon	8 oz	260	35%
Yoplait custard style	6 oz	190	20%
Berries, mixed berries			
Breyers	8 oz	270	30%
Dannon	8 oz	260	35%
Dannon hearty nuts/raisins	8 oz	260	30%
Yoplait custard style	6 oz	180	20%
Black cherry			
Breyers	8 oz	270	30%
Light n' Lively	6 oz	180	20%
Blueberry			
Breyers	8 oz	260	30%
Dannon	8 oz	260	35%
Light n' Lively	6 oz	180	20%
Weight Watchers nonfat	6 oz	150	25%
Yoplait custard style	6 oz	190	20%
Yoplait original	6 oz	190	25%

Yogurt *(continued)*

FOOD / BRAND NAME	SERVING	CALORIES	CALCIUM % U.S. RDA
Boysenberry (Yoplait original)	6 oz	190	25%
Cherry/almonds (Yoplait breakfast)	6 oz	210	50%
Cherry (Dannon)	8 oz	260	35%
Cherry (Yoplait original)	6 oz	190	25%
Cherries jubilee (Yoplait YoCreme)	5 oz	220	20%
Citrus fruits (Yoplait breakfast)	6 oz	250	25%
Coffee (Dannon)	8 oz	200	35%
Lemon			
Dannon	8 oz	200	35%
Weight Watchers nonfat	6 oz	150	25%
Yoplait custard style	6 oz	190	20%
Yoplait original	6 oz	190	25%
Orchard fruit			
Dannon hearty nuts/raisins	8 oz	260	30%
Yoplait breakfast	6 oz	230	20%
Peach			
Breyers	8 oz	270	30%
Dannon	8 oz	260	35%
Yoplait original	6 oz	190	25%
Pina Colada			
Dannon	8 oz	260	35%
Yoplait original	6 oz	190	25%
Pineapple			
Breyers	8 oz	270	30%
Light n' Lively	6 oz	180	20%
Yoplait original	6 oz	190	25%
Plain			
Breyers	8 oz	190	40%
Dannon	8 oz	150	40%
Dannon, nonfat	8 oz	110	45%
Weight Watchers nonfat	6 oz	90	30%
Yoplait extra mild	8 oz	160	40%
Yoplait original	6 oz	130	30%
Raspberry, red raspberry			
Breyers	8 oz	260	30%
Dannon	8 oz	260	35%

Yogurt, raspberry *(continued)*

FOOD / BRAND NAME	SERVING	CALORIES	CALCIUM % U.S. RDA
Dannon fresh flavors	8 oz	200	40%
Light n' Lively	6 oz	170	20%
Yoplait custard style	6 oz	190	20%
Yoplait original	6 oz	190	25%
Raspberries & cream			
Yoplait YoCreme	5 oz	230	20%
Strawberry			
Breyers	8 oz	270	30%
Dannon	8 oz	260	35%
Dannon fresh flavors	8 oz	200	40%
Light n' Lively	6 oz	180	20%
Weight Watchers nonfat	6 oz	150	25%
Yoplait custard	6 oz	190	20%
Yoplait original	6 oz	190	25%
Strawberry banana			
Breyers	6 oz	200	20%
Dannon	8 oz	260	35%
Dannon fresh flavors	8 oz	200	40%
Light 'n Lively	6 oz	200	20%
Yoplait breakfast	6 oz	240	50%
Strawberry w/almonds			
Yoplait breakfast	6 oz	210	50%
Strawberries romanoff			
Yoplait YoCreme	5 oz	220	20%
Sunrise peach (Yoplait breakfast)	6 oz	230	50%
Tropical fruits (Yoplait breakfast)	6 oz	230	50%
Vanilla, vanilla bean			
Breyers	8 oz	230	35%
Dannon fresh flavors	8 oz	200	40%
Dannon hearty nuts/raisins	8 oz	260	30%
Weight Watchers nonfat	6 oz	150	25%
Yoplait custard style	6 oz	180	25%

Fresh fish

Clams, raw, meat only	3 oz	65	6%
Oysters, raw, medium selects (13-19)	1 cup	160	22%

Frozen Foods

FOOD / BRAND NAME	SERVING	CALORIES	CALCIUM % U.S. RDA
Breakfast products			
Eggs, scrambled w/sausage (Swanson)	6 1/4 oz	430	8%
French toast (Aunt Jemima)	2 slices	170	8%
cinnamon swirl (Aunt Jemima)	2 slices	210	8%
w/sausages (Swanson Great Starts)	6 1/2 oz	460	10%
Omelets			
Spanish style (Swanson)	7 3/4 oz	250	8%
Spanish style w/hash browns (Swanson)	8 oz	250	10%
w/cheese sauce & ham (Swanson)	7 oz	400	25%
Pancake batter (4" pancake)			
blueberry (Aunt Jemima)	3	210	4%
buttermilk (Aunt Jemima)	3	210	8%
plain (Aunt Jemima)	3	210	4%
Pancakes			
& blueberry sauce (Swanson)	7 oz	410	6%
buttermilk, 4" (Aunt Jemima)	3	250	6%
original, 4" (Aunt Jemima)	3	260	4%
& sausages (Swanson)	6 oz	470	8%
Waffles			
blueberry			
Aunt Jemima	2	170	10%
Eggo homestyle	1	130	2%
Downyflake	1	170	*
Roman Meal	2	280	4%
buttermilk			
Aunt Jemima	2	170	10%
Downyflake	2	170	*
Eggo	1	120	2%
homestyle (Eggo)	1	120	2%
original (Aunt Jemima)	2	170	10%
raisin (Aunt Jemima)	2	200	10%

* Less than 2% U.S. RDA

Desserts

FOOD / BRAND NAME	SERVING	CALORIES	CALCIUM % U.S. RDA
Desserts			
Cheesecake			
black cherry (Weight Watchers)	3.9 oz	190	8%
strawberry (Weight Watchers)	3.9 oz	180	6%
Ice cream			
banana (Breyers)	4 oz	130	8%
banana split sundae (Breyers)	4 oz	150	8%
butter pecan (Haagen-Dazs)	4 oz	310	8%
buttered pecan (Lady Borden)	$^1/_2$ cup	180	8%
cherry-vanilla (Breyers)	$^1/_2$ cup	140	10%
chocolate			
Breyers	$^1/_2$ cup	160	8%
Haagen-Dazs	4 oz	280	15%
chocolate chip (Breyers)	$^1/_2$ cup	180	10%
chocolate chocolate chip (Haagen-Dazs)	4 oz	310	10%
chocolate choc. mint (Haagen-Dazs)	4 oz	300	10%
chocolate swiss almond (Haagen-Dazs)	4 oz	250	15%
chocolate swirl (Borden)	$^1/_2$ cup	130	6%
coffee (Haagen-Dazs)	4 oz	270	20%
coffee fudge twirl (Breyers)	4 oz	160	10%
cookies & cream (Haagen-Dazs)	4 oz	270	8%
dutch chocolate			
Borden Olde Fashioned	$^1/_2$ cup	130	8%
dutch chocolate almond (Breyers)	4 oz	180	18%
egg nog (Breyers)	$^1/_2$ cup	150	10%
elberta peach (Haagen Dazs)	4 oz	250	20%
honey vanilla (Haagen-Dazs)	4 oz	270	20%
macadamia nut (Haagen-Dazs)	4 oz	260	10%
maple walnut (Haagen-Dazs)	4 oz	320	15%
mocha chip (Haagen-Dazs)	4 oz	270	15%
orange-pineapple (Breyers)	$^1/_2$ cup	140	10%
pumpkin pie (Breyers)	4 oz	150	10%
roasted english walnut (Breyers)	4 oz	170	10%
rum raisin (Haagen-Dazs)	4 oz	260	15%
strawberry			
Borden	$^1/_2$ cup	130	8%
Haagen-Dazs	4 oz	270	15%

Desserts, ice cream *(continued)*

FOOD / BRAND NAME	SERVING	CALORIES	CALCIUM % U.S. RDA
vanilla			
Borden Olde Fashioned	½ cup	130	8%
Breyers	½ cup	150	10%
Haagen-Dazs	4 oz	270	20%
Land O Lakes	4 oz	140	8%
vanilla fudge twirl (Breyers)	½ cup	160	10%
vanilla swiss almond (Haagen-Dazs)	4 oz	340	20%
Ice milk			
caramel nut (Light 'n Lively)	½ cup	120	10%
chocolate			
Borden	½ cup	100	10%
Light n' Lively	½ cup	110	10%
coffee (Light n' Lively)	½ cup	100	10%
heavenly hash (Light n' Lively)	½ cup	120	10%
strawberry (Borden)	½ cup	90	8%
vanilla			
Borden	½ cup	90	10%
Light n' Lively	½ cup	100	10%
vanilla, chocolate & strawberry			
Light n' Lively	½ cup	110	10%
Sherbet and ice			
fruit flavors (Land O Lakes)	4 oz	130	4%
orange (Borden)	½ cup	110	4%
orange & vanilla (Haagen-Dazs)	4 oz	209	10%
pineapple (Sealtest)	½ cup	140	4%
Slices, bars (single serving)			
almond bar, toasted (Good Humor)	1 bar	190	4%
choc. chip pudding bar (Swiss Miss)	1 bar	100	8%
choc. dip froz. dietary dairy dessert			
Weight Watchers	1 bar	100	8%
chocolate malt bar (Good Humor)	1 bar	190	6%
chocolate mint treat (Weight Watchers)	1 bar	60	8%
chocolate pudding bar (Swiss Miss)	1 bar	80	8%
chocolate treat (Weight Watchers)	1 bar	100	15%
double fudge bar (Weight Watchers)	1 bar	60	8%
peach (Dole)	1 bar	90	2%
strawberry (Dole)	1 bar	90	4%

Desserts, ice cream *(continued)*

FOOD / BRAND NAME	SERVING	CALORIES	CALCIUM % U.S. RDA
pudding bars			
chocolate (Swiss Miss)	1 bar	80	8%
chocolate chip (Swiss Miss)	1 bar	100	8%
vanilla (Swiss Miss)	1 bar	90	8%
pudding pops, all flavors (Jell-O)	1 bar	90	8%
pudding stix (Good Humor)	1 bar	90	10%
sandwich bars			
mint (Weight Watchers)	1 bar	130	10%
vanilla (Weight Watchers)	1 bar	130	10%
strawberry vanilla treat			
Weight Watchers	1 bar	100	15%
sundae cone dairy dessert			
Weight Watchers	1 cone	150	8%
vanilla ice cream bar (Good Humor)	1 bar	170	6%
vanilla ice cream sand. (Good Humor)	1 sandwich	170	6%
vanilla ice cream slice (Good Humor)	1 slice	110	6%
vanilla pudding bar (Swiss Miss)	1 bar	90	8%
vanilla sand. bars (Weight Watchers)	1 bar	130	10%
vanilla slice, cal-control (Good Humor)	1 slice	60	6%
Frozen yogurt			
Dannon, frozen Yogurt-on-a-Stick			
all flavors	1 bar	50	6%
Sealtest			
black cherry	$\frac{1}{2}$ cup	100	15%
peach	$\frac{1}{2}$ cup	100	15%
red raspberry	$\frac{1}{2}$ cup	100	15%
strawberry	$\frac{1}{2}$ cup	100	15%
Yoplait soft			
banana/raspberry	3 fl oz	90	6%
mixed berry	3 fl oz	90	8%
Entrees: beef, pork and veal			
Beans and frankfurters			
Banquet dinners	10 oz	510	10%
Swanson	12 $\frac{1}{2}$ oz	550	10%
Beef oriental w/vegetables & rice			
Weight Watchers	10 oz	260	8%

Frozen entrees: beef, pork and veal *(continued)*

FOOD / BRAND NAME	SERVING	CALORIES	CALCIUM % U.S. RDA
Beef pepper steak (Armour Classic Lite)	10 $^1/_2$ oz	290	6%
Beef salisbury steak romana			
Weight Watchers	8 $^3/_4$ oz	300	15%
Beefsteak, chopped (Weight Watchers)	9 $^3/_4$ oz	290	6%
Beef Stroganoff (Le Menu)	10 oz	430	15%
w/parsley noodles (Stouffer's)	9 $^3/_4$ oz	410	6%
Beef w/gravy (Banquet American			
Favorites dinners)	10 oz	345	6%
Beef ribs, boneless			
Armour Dinner Classics	10 $^1/_2$ oz	420	8%
Chopped sirloin beef (Swanson)	11 $^1/_2$ oz	370	10%
Creamed chipped beef (Stouffer's)	5 $^1/_2$ oz	240	10%
Ham & asparagus crepes (Stouffer's)	6 $^1/_4$ oz	310	15%
Meat loaf (Banquet dinners)	11 oz	440	6%
Pepper steak, beef			
Armour Classic Lite	10 $^1/_2$ oz	290	6%
Ribs, beef, boneless			
Armour Dinner Classics	10 $^1/_2$ oz	420	8%
Salisbury steak (Armour dinner classics)	11 oz	460	6%
Salisbury steak			
w/Italian style sauce & vegetables			
Stouffer's Lean Cuisine	9 $^1/_2$ oz	270	15%
w/onion gravy (Weight Watchers)	8 $^3/_4$ oz	300	15%
Sirloin of beef, chopped & formed			
Weight Watchers	13 oz	410	10%
Sirloin tips (Armour Dinner Classics)	11 oz	340	15%
Stuffed green peppers (Weight Watchers)	11 $^3/_4$ oz	300	4%
Swedish meatballs			
Armour Dinner Classics	12 $^1/_2$ oz	480	10%
w/parsley noodles (Stouffer's)	11 oz	470	6%
Sweet & sour chicken			
Armour Classics Lite	10 $^1/_2$ oz	250	4%
Veal parmigiana			
Armour Dinner Classics	10 $^3/_4$ oz	400	10%
Swanson	12 $^1/_4$ oz	460	15%
Swanson Hungry Man	18 $^1/_4$ oz	630	15%
Veal patty parmigiana (Weight Watchers)	8 $^7/_{16}$ oz	220	20%

Entrees: cheese combinations

FOOD / BRAND NAME	SERVING	CALORIES	CALCIUM % U.S. RDA
Entrees: cheese combinations			
Beef/cheese enchilada w/rice & beans			
Van de Kamp's Mex. Classic Comb.	14 3/4 oz	540	35%
Cheese cannelloni w/tomato sauce			
Stouffer's Lean Cuisine	9 1/8 oz	270	30%
Cheese enchilada(s)			
Van de Kamp's Mexican Holiday	7 1/2 oz	270	30%
Van de Kamp's Mexican Holiday	(4) 8 1/2 oz	370	45%
Cheese enchiladas ranchero			
Van de Kamp's Mexican Classic	5 1/2 oz	250	25%
Cheese enchilada w/rice & beans			
Van de Kamp's Mex. Classic Comb.	14 3/4 oz	620	50%
Cheese ravioli (Weight Watchers)	9 oz	300	30%
Cheese souffle (Stouffer's)	7 5/8 oz	480	40%
Crepes, ham & asparagus (Stouffer's)	6 1/4 oz	310	15%
Crepes, ham & swiss cheese (Stouffer's)	7 1/2 oz	410	40%
Crepes, spinach w/cheddar cheese sauce			
Stouffer's	9 1/2 oz	420	30%
Cheese stuffed pasta shells w/meat sauce			
Stouffer's	9 oz	320	40%
Cheese stuffed shells (Le Menu Light)	10 oz	280	15%
Eggplant parmigiana			
Buitoni	12 oz	430	30%
Mrs. Paul's	5 1/2 oz	270	10%
Italian cheese lasagne (Weight Watchers)	12 oz	360	40%
Lasagna			
beef & mushroom			
Van de Kamp's Italian Classics	11 oz	430	45%
creamy spinach			
Van de Kamp's Italian Classics	11 oz	400	50%
deep dish (Buitoni)	11 oz	390	25%
florentine (Buitoni)	9 1/2 oz	480	50%
florentine (Light & Elegant)	11 1/4 oz	280	28%
Italian cheese (Weight Watchers)	12 oz	360	40%
Italian sausage			
Van de Kamp's Italian Classics	11 oz	440	45%
Stouffer's, 21 oz	10 1/2 oz	370	25%

Frozen entrees: cheese combinations, lasagna *(continued)*

FOOD / BRAND NAME	SERVING	CALORIES	CALCIUM % U.S. RDA
w/meat sauce (Buitoni)	14 oz	540	35%
w/meat sauce			
Green Giant Baked Entree	12 oz	490	50%
Green Giant Baked Entree	10 $^1/_2$ oz	430	45%
w/meat (Swanson Hungry Man dinner)	18 $^3/_4$ oz	740	30%
vegetable			
Le Menu	11 oz	360	20%
Weight Watchers	12 oz	360	15%
zucchini (Stouffer's Lean Cuisine)	11 oz	260	30%
Macaroni & cheese			
Banquet Casserole	8 oz	344	21%
Banquet Family Favorites Dinners	10 oz	415	27%
Light & Elegant	9 oz	300	32%
Swanson pot pie	7 oz	220	15%
Swanson entree	12 oz	390	25%
Swanson dinner	12 $^1/_4$ oz	380	20%
Manicotti in sauce (Buitoni)	13 oz	420	30%
Meat ravioli parmesan (Buitoni)	12 oz	520	30%
Omelet w/cheese sauce ham (Swanson)	7 oz	400	20%
Pizza *(see listings page 195)*			
Quiche			
ham (Land O' Lakes)	4 $^1/_3$ oz	230	25%
spinach & onion			
Pour-A-Quiche, Land O Lakes	4 $^1/_3$ oz	220	30%
3-cheese/bacon & onion			
Pour-A-Quiche, Land O Lakes	4 $^1/_3$ oz	230	30%
Round cheese ravioli (Buitoni)	5 $^1/_2$ oz	310	30%
Seafood cannelloni (On-Cor Lite)	8 oz	210	25%
Seafood newburg			
Armour Dinner Classics	11 $^1/_2$ oz	300	10%
Spinach & cheese stuffed shells (Buitoni)	5 $^1/_2$ oz	160	20%
Stuffed shells w/sauce (Buitoni)	10 oz	350	45%
Tortellini guido (Buitoni)	10 oz	380	40%
Vegetable manicotti marinara			
On-Cor Lite	8 oz	180	25%
Spinach crepes w/cheddar cheese sauce			
Stouffer's	9 $^1/_2$ oz	420	30%

Frozen entrees: cheese combinations *(continued)*

FOOD / BRAND NAME	SERVING	CALORIES	CALCIUM % U.S. RDA
Veal, veal patty parmigiana			
Swanson	12 1/4 oz	460	15%
Swanson Hungry Man dinner	18 1/4 oz	630	15%
Weight Watchers	8 7/16 oz	220	20%
Welsh rarebit (Stouffer's)	5 oz	360	40%

Entrees: fish

FOOD / BRAND NAME	SERVING	CALORIES	CALCIUM % U.S. RDA
Baby bay shrimp (Armour Classics Lite)	10 1/2 oz	250	15%
Comb. seafood platter (Mrs. Paul's)	9 oz	590	8%
Crabmeat, snow (Wakefield)	3 oz	60	2%
Crabs, deviled (Mrs. Paul's)	1 (3 oz)	190	8%
Crab miniatures, deviled (Mrs. Paul's)	3 1/2 oz	250	8%
Crown of flounder divan (Mrs. Paul's)	9 oz	200	8%
Filet of fish, au gratin (Weight Watchers)	9 1/4 oz	220	15%
Filet of fish divan			
Stouffer's Lean Cuisine	12 3/8 oz	270	20%
Filet of fish florentine			
Stouffer's Lean Cuisine	9 oz	240	15%
Fish (Banquet Platters)	8 3/4 oz	445	8%
Fish fillets, supreme light batter			
Mrs. Paul's	3 5/8 oz	220	6%
Fish florentine			
Mrs. Paul's light seafood	9 oz	210	30%
Fish florentine, filet of			
Stouffer's Lean Cuisine	9 oz	240	15%
Fish & pasta florentine (Mrs. Paul's)	9 1/2 oz	240	25%
Fish mornay w/broccoli			
Mrs. Paul's light seafood	10 oz	280	10%
Fish parmesan (Mrs. Paul's)	5 oz	220	10%
Fish sticks (Mrs. Paul's)	4 sticks	200	2%
French fried scallops (Mrs. Paul's)	3 1/2 oz	230	6%
Italian style fish fillet in tomato sauce w/cheese (Weight Watchers)	9 oz	180	15%
Lobster newburg (Stouffer's)	6 1/2 oz	360	10%
Scallops & shrimp mariner w/rice			
Stouffer's	10 1/4 oz	390	15%

Frozen entrees: fish *(continued)*

FOOD / BRAND NAME	SERVING	CALORIES	CALCIUM % U.S. RDA
Scallops, french fried (Mrs. Paul's)	3 1/2 oz	230	4%
Seafoods w/natural herbs			
Armour Classics Lite	10 1/2 oz	220	15%
Seafood newburg			
Armour Dinner Classics	11 1/2 oz	300	10%
Shrimp creole w/rice			
Green Giant Boil 'n Bag	9 oz	230	5%
Shrimp marinara (Buitoni)	11 oz	210	6%
Snow crabmeat (Wakefield)	3 oz	60	2%
Stuffed flounder (Le Menu)	10 1/2 oz	350	8%
Tuna noodle casserole (Stouffer's)	5 3/4 oz	190	8%
Tuna pasta casserole			
Mrs. Paul'sl light seafood	11 oz	290	35%
Tuna pie (Banquet)	8 oz	510	10%

Entrees: Mexican

Bean & beef burrito (Swanson)	15 1/4 oz	720	15%
Beef & bean burritos w/chili salsa			
Van de Kamp's	6 oz	280	5%
Beef/cheese enchilada w/rice & beans			
(Van de Kamp's Mex Classic Comb)	14 3/4 oz	540	35%
Beef enchilada dinner (Van de			
Kamp's Mexican Holiday)	12 oz	390	19%
Beef enchilada(s)			
Swanson Dinner	13 3/4 oz	480	20%
Van de Kamp's Mexican Holiday	7 1/2 oz	250	15%
Van de Kamp's Mexican Holiday	(4) 8 1/2 oz	340	25%
Van de Kamp's Mexican Holiday	(2) 5 1/2 oz	226	10%
Weight Watchers, Ranchero	9 1/2 oz	310	25%
Beef enchilada, shredded (Van de Kamp's)	5 1/2 oz	180	20%
Beef enchilada, shredded w/rice &			
corn (Van de Kamp's Mexican			
Classic Combinations)	14 3/4 oz	490	15%
Beef taquitos, shredded w/guacamole			
Van de Kamp's	8 oz	490	10%
Beef tostada supreme (Van de Kamp's)	8 1/2 oz	530	35%

Frozen entrees: Mexican *(continued)*

FOOD / BRAND NAME	SERVING	CALORIES	CALCIUM % U.S. RDA
Burritos			
bean & beef (Swanson)	15 1/4 oz	720	15%
green chili beef/bean (Van de Kamp's)	5 oz	330	10%
red chili beef/bean (Van de Kamp's)	5 oz	320	10%
sirloin, grande (Van de Kamp's)	11 oz	440	20%
w/rice & corn, grande (Van de Kamp's Mexican Classics)	14 3/4 oz	530	20%
Cheese enchilada dinner (Van de Kamp's Mexican Holiday)	12 oz	450	20%
Cheese enchilada ranchero			
Van de Kamp's Mexican Classics	5 1/2 oz	250	25%
Cheese enchilada(s)			
Van de Kamp's Mexican Holiday	7 1/2 oz	270	30%
Van de Kamp's Mexican Holiday	(4) 8 1/2 oz	370	45%
Cheese enchilada w/rice & beans			
Van de Kamp's Mex. Classic Comb.	14 3/4 oz	620	50%
Chicken enchilada(s)			
Van de Kamp's Mexican Holiday	7 1/2 oz	250	20%
Chicken enchiladas suiza			
Van de Kamp's Mexican Classics	5 1/2 oz	220	30%
Weight Watchers	8 1/2 oz	310	25%
Chicken suiza w/rice & beans (Van de Kamp's Mexican Classic Comb.)	14 3/4 oz	550	45%
Chili con carne w/beans (Stouffer's)	8 3/4 oz	280	8%
Enchilada(s)			
beef/cheese, w/rice & beans			
Van de Kamp's Mex. Classic Comb.	14 3/4 oz	540	35%
beef			
Swanson Dinner	13 3/4 oz	480	20%
Van de Kamp's Mexican Holiday	7 1/2 oz	250	15%
Van de Kamp's Mexican Holiday	(4) 8 1/2 oz	340	25%
Weight Watchers, Ranchero	9 1/8 oz	310	25%
beef, shredded (Van de Kamp's)	5 1/2 oz	180	20%
beef, shredded w/rice & corn			
Van de Kamp's Mexican Classic Comb.	14 3/4 oz	490	15%

Frozen entrees: Mexican, enchiladas *(continued)*

FOOD / BRAND NAME	SERVING	CALORIES	CALCIUM % U.S. RDA
cheese			
Van de Kamp's Mexican Holiday	7 $\frac{1}{2}$ oz	270	30%
Van de Kamp's Mexican Holiday	(4) 8 $\frac{1}{2}$ oz	370	45%
cheese ranchero			
Van de Kamp's	5 $\frac{1}{2}$ oz	250	25%
Weight Watchers	8 $\frac{1}{8}$ oz	370	45%
ranchero w/rice & beans (Van de Kamp's Mexican Classic Comb.	14 $\frac{3}{4}$ oz	620	50%
chicken			
Van de Kamp's Mexican Holiday	7 $\frac{1}{2}$ oz	250	20%
chicken suiza			
Van de Kamp's Mexican Classics	5 $\frac{1}{2}$ oz	220	30%
Weight Watchers	8 $\frac{1}{2}$ oz	310	25%
dinner, beef enchilada (Van de Kamp's Mexican Holiday)	12 oz	390	20%
dinner, cheese enchilada (Van de Kamp's Mexican Holiday)	12 oz	450	20%
grande burrito w/rice & corn (Van de Kamp's Mexican Classic Comb.)	14 $\frac{3}{4}$ oz	530	20%
Mexican style			
Swanson Hungry Man dinner	20 $\frac{1}{4}$ oz	750	30%
Mexican style dinner			
Van de Kamp's Mexican Holiday	11 $\frac{1}{2}$ oz	420	15%
shredded beef enchiladas			
Van de Kamp's Mexican Classic	5 $\frac{1}{2}$ oz	180	20%
shredded beef enchilada w/rice & corn			
Van de Kamp's Mexican Classic	14 $\frac{3}{4}$ oz	490	20%
shredded beef taquitos w/guacamole			
Van de Kamp's	8 oz	490	10%
sirloin burrito grande (Van de Kamp's)	11 oz	440	20%
Frozen entrees: pasta			
Baked cheese ravioli (Weight Watchers)	9 oz	300	30%
Baked shells w/sauce (Buitoni)	10 $\frac{1}{2}$ oz	320	10%
Baked ziti (Buitoni)	10 $\frac{1}{2}$ oz	360	15%
Beef & mushroom lasagna			
Van de Kamp's Italian Classics	11 oz	430	45%

Frozen entrees: pasta *(continued)*

FOOD / BRAND NAME	SERVING	CALORIES	CALCIUM % U.S. RDA
Beef & pork cannelloni w/mornay sauce			
Stouffer's Lean Cuisine	9 5/8 oz	270	20%
Beef & spinach stuffed pasta shells			
w/tomato sauce (Stouffer's)	9 oz	300	15%
Broccoli stuffed shells (Buitoni)	5 oz	150	15%
Cheese cannelloni w/tomato sauce			
Stouffer's Lean Cuisine	9 1/8 oz	270	30%
Cheese ravioli			
Buitoni, 40 ct	3 3/4 oz	260	10%
Weight Watchers	9 oz	300	30%
parmesan (Buitoni)	12 oz	440	15%
Cheese stuffed pasta shells w/meat sauce			
Stouffer's	9 oz	340	40%
Chicken stuffed pasta shells			
w/cheese sauce (Stouffer's)	9 oz	420	35%
Creamy spinach lasagna			
Van de Kamp's Italian Classics)	11 oz	400	50%
Deep dish lasagna (Buitoni)	11 oz	390	25%
Deep dish lasagna w/meat sauce (Buitoni)	10 1/2 oz	400	10%
Fetuccine			
alfredo (Buitoni)	10 oz	440	50%
carbonara (Buitoni)	10 oz	440	40%
primavera (Buitoni)	10 oz	449	10%
Italian cheese lasagne (Weight Watchers)	12 oz	360	40%
Italian sausage lasagna			
Van de Kamp's Italian Classics	11 oz	440	47%
Jumbo manicotti (Buitoni)	6 oz	270	35%
Lasagna			
Banquet Extra Helping Dinners	16 1/2 oz	645	32%
Stouffer's, 21 oz	10 1/2 oz	370	25%
Swanson	13 oz	420	15%
beef & mushroom			
Van de Kamp's Italian Classics	11 oz	430	45%
creamy spinach			
Van de Kamp's Italian Classics	11 oz	400	50%
deep dish (Buitoni)	11 oz	390	25%
deep dish, w/meat sauce (Buitoni)	10 1/2 oz	400	10%

193

Frozen entrees: pasta, lasagne *(continued)*

FOOD / BRAND NAME	SERVING	CALORIES	CALCIUM % U.S. RDA
florentine			
Buitoni	9 1/2 oz	480	50%
Light & Elegant	11 1/4 oz	280	28%
Italian cheese (Weight Watchers)	12 oz	360	40%
Italian sausage			
Van de Kamp's Italian Classics	11 oz	440	45%
w/meat (Swanson Hungry Man)	18 3/4 oz	730	30%
w/meat sauce			
Buitoni	14 oz	540	35%
Green Giant Baked Entree	12 oz	490	50%
Weight Watchers	11 oz	330	25%
vegetable			
Le Menu	11 oz	400	25%
Stouffer's single serving or 21 oz	10 1/2 oz	450	50%
vegetable alfredo			
On-Cor Lite	8 oz	240	20%
Weight Watchers	12 oz	360	15%
zucchini (Stouffer's Lean Cuisine)	11 oz	260	30%
Macaroni & beef w/tomatoes (Stouffer's)	11 1/2 oz	360	6%
Macaroni & cheese			
Banquet Casserole	8 oz	344	21%
Banquet Family Favorites Dinners	10 oz	415	27%
Light & Elegant	9 oz	300	32%
Swanson	7 oz	210	20%
Swanson	12 oz	390	25%
Swanson Dinner	12 1/4 oz	380	20%
Manicotti in sauce (Buitoni)	13 oz	420	30%
Meat ravioli, 40 ct (Buitoni)	3 3/4 oz	265	8%
Meat ravioli parmesan (Buitoni)	12 oz	520	30%
Round cheese ravioli (Buitoni)	5 1/2 oz	310	30%
Seafood cannelloni (On-Cor Lite)	8 oz	210	25%
Spaghetti w/beef & mushroom sauce			
Stouffer's Lean Cusine	11 1/2 oz	280	6%
Spaghetti w/meat sauce			
Stouffer's	14 oz	440	10%
Weight Watchers	10 1/2 oz	280	6%

Frozen entrees: pasta *(continued)*

FOOD / BRAND NAME	SERVING	CALORIES	CALCIUM % U.S. RDA
Tortellini w/meat			
Armour Dinner Classics Lite	10 oz	250	20%
Tortellini guido (Buitoni)	10 oz	380	40%
Vegetable lasagna (Le Menu)	11 oz	360	20%
Vegetable lasagna			
Stouffer's single serving or 21 oz	$10\frac{1}{2}$ oz	450	50%
Vegetable lasagne alfredo (On-Cor Lite)	8 oz	240	20%
Vegetable manicotti marinara			
On-Cor Lite	8 oz	180	25%
Ziti, baked (Buitoni)	$10\frac{1}{2}$ oz	350	15%
Ziti macaroni w/meat, tomato sauce			
& cheese (Weight Watchers)	$11\frac{1}{4}$ oz	290	25%
Zucchini lasagna (Stouffer's Lean Cuisine)	11 oz	260	30%

Entrees: pizza

FOOD / BRAND NAME	SERVING	CALORIES	CALCIUM % U.S. RDA
Canadian/Canadian style bacon			
Celeste, 19 oz	$\frac{1}{4}$ pizza	340	25%
Celeste, $7\frac{3}{4}$ oz	1 pizza	550	40%
Totino's My Classic	$\frac{1}{4}$ pizza	320	20%
Totino's Party	$\frac{1}{3}$ pizza	230	20%
Cheese			
Buitoni, instant	2 oz	130	10%
Celeste, $6\frac{1}{2}$ oz	1 pizza	500	30%
Celeste, $17\frac{3}{4}$ oz	$\frac{1}{4}$ pizza	330	20%
Stouffer's French Bread	$5\frac{3}{16}$ oz	340	20%
Totino's My Classic, deluxe	$\frac{1}{4}$ pizza	350	30%
Totino's Party	$\frac{1}{3}$ pizza	250	15%
Weight Watchers	6 oz	350	35%
Deluxe			
Celeste, $8\frac{1}{4}$ oz	1 pizza	600	30%
Celeste, $22\frac{1}{4}$ oz	$\frac{1}{4}$ pizza	390	20%
Stouffer's French Bread	$6\frac{3}{16}$ oz	430	20%
Totino's My Classic, cheese	$\frac{1}{4}$ pizza	350	30%
Totino's My Classic, combination	$\frac{1}{4}$ pizza	460	25%
Weight Watchers combination	$7\frac{1}{4}$ oz	340	25%
Hamburger			
Totino's Party	$\frac{1}{3}$ pizza	230	20%

Frozen pizza, hamburger *(continued)*

FOOD / BRAND NAME	SERVING	CALORIES	CALCIUM % U.S. RDA
Stouffer's French Bread	6 1/8 oz	410	20%
Instant cheese (Buitoni)	2 oz	130	10%
Mexican style (Totino's Party)	1/3 pizza	240	10%
Nacho (Totino's Party)	1/3 pizza	230	20%
Pepperoni			
Celeste, 6 3/4 oz	1 pizza	580	25%
Celeste, 19 oz	1/4 pizza	370	25%
Fox deluxe	1/3 pizza	170	6%
Stouffer's French Bread	5 5/8 oz	390	20%
Totino's My Classic, deluxe	1/4 pizza	410	25%
Totino's Party	1/3 pizza	260	10%
Weight Watchers	6 1/4 oz	370	10%
Sausage			
Celeste, 7 1/2 oz	1 pizza	580	30%
Celeste, 20 oz	1/4 pizza	390	25%
Stouffer's French Bread	6 oz	420	20%
Totino's My Classic, deluxe	1/4 pizza	440	25%
Totino's Party	1/3 pizza	270	20%
Sausage & mushroom			
Celeste, 8 1/2 oz	1 pizza	600	30%
Celeste, 22 1/2 oz	1/4 pizza	410	25%
Stouffer's French Bread	6 1/4 oz	400	10%
Sausage & pepperoni			
Buitoni, 6-slice	4 oz	220	20%
Totino's Party	1/3 pizza	270	10%
Suprema (Celeste), 9 oz	1 pizza	690	35%
23 oz	1/4 pizza	410	25%
Veal sausage (Weight Watchers)	6 3/4 oz	350	25%

Entrees: poultry

Breast of chicken parmigiana (Le Menu)	11 1/2 oz	380	15%
Chicken a la king			
Le Menu dinner	10 1/4 oz	330	6%
Weight Watchers	9 oz	230	20%
w/rice (Stouffer's)	9 1/2 oz	320	8%
Chicken & noodles (Green Giant)	9 oz	370	15%

Frozen entrees: poultry *(continued)*

FOOD / BRAND NAME	SERVING	CALORIES	CALCIUM % U.S. RDA
Chicken & vegetables w/vermicelli			
Stouffer's Lean Cuisine	$12\,^3/_4$ oz	270	10%
Chicken cacciatore			
Stouffer's Lean Cuisine	$10\,^7/_8$ oz	280	4%
Weight Watchers	$10\,^1/_2$ oz	290	4%
Chicken cordon bleu (Le Menu Dinner)	11 oz	470	10%
Chicken, creamed (Stouffer's)	$6\,^1/_2$ oz	320	6%
Chicken crepes w/mushroom sauce			
Stouffer's	$8\,^1/_4$ oz	370	15%
Chicken divan (Stouffer's)	$8\,^1/_2$ oz	350	20%
Chicken, escalloped & noodles (Stouffer's)	$5\,^3/_4$ oz	260	4%
Chicken breast florentine			
Le Menu Dinner	$12\,^1/_2$ oz	480	15%
Chicken florentine (Le Menu Dinner)	$12\,^1/_2$ oz	480	15%
Chicken fricassee			
Armour Dinner Classics	$11^3/_4$ oz	340	10%
Chicken in cheese sauce (Light & Elegant)	$8\,^3/_4$ oz	295	20%
Chicken parmigiana, breast of (Le Menu)	$11^1/_2$ oz	380	15%
Chicken patty parmigiana			
Weight Watchers	$8\,^1/_{16}$ oz	280	20%
Chicken pie (Stouffer's)	10 oz	530	8%
Creamed chicken (Stouffer's)	$6\,^1/_2$ oz	320	6%
Escalloped chicken & noodles (Stouffer's)	$5\,^3/_4$ oz	260	4%
Fried chicken			
Banquet Extra Helping Dinners	16 oz	560	6%
Turkey breast, stuffed (Weight Watchers)	$8\,^1/_2$ oz	260	6%
Turkey casserole w/gravy & dressing			
Stouffer's	$9\,^3/_4$ oz	380	10%
Turkey divan (Le Menu Light Style)	10 oz	280	10%
Turkey pie (Stouffer's)	10 oz	540	8%
Turkey tetrazzini (Stouffer's)	6 oz	230	6%
Vegetables			
Asparagus			
cuts (Birds Eye)	3.3 oz	25	2%
spears (Birds Eye)	3.3 oz	25	2%

Frozen vegetables *(continued)*

FOOD / BRAND NAME	SERVING	CALORIES	CALCIUM % U.S. RDA
Broccoli			
& water chestnuts (Birds Eye)	3.3 oz	50	6%
baby spears (Birds Eye)	3.3 oz	30	4%
chopped (Birds Eye)	3.3 oz	25	4%
cuts (Birds Eye)	3.3 oz	25	6%
cuts (Green Giant polybag)	$^1/_2$ cup	16	2%
Fanfare (Green Giant Harvest			
Get Togethers)	$^1/_2$ cup	70	2%
florets (Birds Eye)	3.3 oz	25	4%
in cheddar cheese sauce (Stouffer's)	4 $^1/_2$ oz	150	15%
minispears (Green Giant Frozen			
Like Fresh)	$^1/_2$ cup	16	0%
spears (Birds Eye)	3.3 oz	25	4%
spears (Green Giant Harvest Fresh)	$^1/_2$ cup	30	2%
spears/butter sauce (Green Giant)	$^1/_2$ cup	45	2%
w/cheese in pastry (Pepperidge Farm)	1	250	6%
w/cheese sauce (Birds Eye)	5 oz	120	10%
w/cheese sauce (Green Giant)	$^1/_2$ cup	70	6%
w/creamy Italian cheese sauce			
Birds Eye	4 $^1/_2$ oz	90	10%
w/white cheddar cheese sauce			
Green Giant	$^1/_2$ cup	60	6%
Broccoli combinations			
broccoli & cauliflower w/creamy			
Italian cheese sauce (Birds Eye)	4.5 oz	90	8%
broccoli & cauliflower w/red peppers			
Birds Eye	3.3 oz	25	2%
broccoli, carrots & pasta twists			
Birds Eye	3.3 oz	90	4%
broccoli, carrots fanfare			
Green Giant Valley Combination	$^1/_2$ cup	20	2%
broccoli, cauliflower & carrots			
w/cheese sauce (Birds Eye)	5 oz	100	8%
broccoli, cauliflower, carrots			
w/cheese sauce (Green Giant)	$^1/_2$ cup	70	6%
broccoli cauliflower medley			
Green Giant Valley Combination	$^1/_2$ cup	60	2%

Frozen vegetables: broccoli combinations *(continued)*

FOOD / BRAND NAME	SERVING	CALORIES	CALCIUM % U.S. RDA
broccoli, cauliflower, supreme			
Green Giant Valley Combination	$^1/_2$ cup	18	2%
broccoli/rice 'n, flavored cheese sauce			
Green Giant Rice Originals	$^1/_2$ cup	120	4%
Brussels sprouts			
Birds Eye	3.3 oz	35	2%
Green Giant polybag	$^1/_2$ cup	30	2%
baby, w/cheese sauce (Birds Eye)	4.5 oz	110	8%
/butter sauce (Green Giant)	$^1/_2$ cup	60	2%
Carrot(s)			
crinkle cutter/butter sauce (Green Giant)	$^1/_2$ cup	80	2%
whole baby (Birds Eye)	3.3 oz	40	2%
Carrot combinations			
w/pasta twists/(Birds Eye)	3.3 oz	90	4%
fanfare (Green Giant polybag)	$^1/_2$ cup	25	2%
w/cauliflower & cheese sauce			
Birds Eye	5 oz	100	8%
w/cauliflower & cheese sauce			
Green Giant	$^1/_2$ cup	70	6%
Cauliflower (Birds Eye)	3.3 oz	25	2%
cuts (Green Giant polybag)	$^1/_2$ cup	12	2%
in butter sauce (Green Giant)	$^1/_2$ cup	30	2%
in white cheddar cheese sauce			
(Green Giant)	$^1/_2$ cup	60	6%
w/cheese sauce (Birds Eye)	5 oz	110	8%
Cauliflower combinations			
broccoli, cauliflower & carrots			
w/cheese sauce (Birds Eye)	5 oz	100	8%
broccoli, cauliflower, carrots			
w/cheese sauce (Green Giant)	$^1/_2$ cup	70	6%
broccoli, cauliflower medley			
Green Giant Valley Combination	$^1/_2$ cup	60	2%
broccoli, cauliflower supreme			
Green Giant polybag	$^1/_2$ cup	18	2%
cauliflower, carrots/snow pea pods			
Birds Eye	3.2 oz	30	2%

Frozen vegetables *(continued)*

FOOD / BRAND NAME	SERVING	CALORIES	CALCIUM % U.S. RDA
Chopped collard greens (PictSweet)	3.2 oz	25	20%
Chopped mustard greens (PictSweet)	3.2 oz	20	10%
Chopped turnip greens (PictSweet)	3.2 oz	20	10%
Collard greens, chopped (PictSweet)	3.2 oz	25	20%
Corn			
big ears on the cob (Birds Eye)	1 ear	160	*
little ears on the cob (Birds Eye)	2 ears	130	*
sweet (Birds Eye)	3.3 oz	80	*
Corn, green beans & pasta curls			
Birds Eye	3.3 oz	110	6%
Eggplant parmigiana			
Buitoni	12 oz	430	30%
Mrs. Paul's	5 1/2 oz	270	10%
Green beans (Green Giant polybag)	1/2 cup	20	2%
cut (Birds Eye)	3 oz	25	4%
cut (Green Giant Harvest Fresh)	1/2 cup	20	2%
french cut (Birds Eye)	3 oz	25	4%
french style/butter sauce (Green Giant)	1/2 cup	40	2%
in cream sauce w/mushrooms			
Green Giant	1/2 cup	80	4%
Italian (Birds Eye)	3 oz	30	4%
Greens			
collard greens, chopped (PictSweet)	3.2 oz	25	10%
mustard greens, chopped (PictSweet)	3.2 oz	20	10%
turnip greens, chopped (PictSweet)	3.2 oz	20	10%
Italian blend white rice & spinach/cheese			
sauce (Green Giant Rice Orig)	1/2 cup	170	6%
Lima beans			
Fordhook (Birds Eye)	3.3 oz	100	2%
Green Giant Harvest Fresh	1/2 cup	70	2%
baby (Birds Eye)	3.3 oz	130	4%
/butter sauce (Green Giant)	1/2 cup	120	2%
Mexican style vegetables			
Green Giant Valley Combination	1/2 cup	150	6%

* Less than 2% U.S. RDA

Frozen vegetables *(continued)*

FOOD / BRAND NAME	SERVING	CALORIES	CALCIUM % U.S. RDA
Mixed vegetables			
Green Giant Harvest Fresh	$1/2$ cup	45	2%
/butter sauce (Green Giant)	$1/2$ cup	80	2%
w/onion sauce (Birds Eye)	2 6 oz	100	4%
Mustard greens, chopped (PictSweet)	3.2 oz	20	10%
Okra			
cut (Birds Eye)	3.3 oz	25	8%
whole (Birds Eye)	3.3 oz	30	8%
whole (PictSweet)	3.3 oz	30	8%
Onions			
small whole (Birds Eye)	4 oz	40	4%
small w/cream sauce (Birds Eye)	3 oz	110	6%
Peas			
& pearl onions w/cheese sauce			
(Birds Eye)	5 oz	140	8%
early June (Green Giant)	$1/2$ cup	60	2%
green (Birds Eye)	3.3 oz	80	2%
in cream sauce (Green Giant)	$1/2$ cup	100	4%
w/cream sauce (Birds Eye)	2.6 oz	120	4%
Potatoes			
au gratin (Stouffer's)	3.8 oz	120	8%
scalloped (Stouffer's)	4 oz	110	8%
and sweet peas in bacon cream			
sauce (Green Giant)	$1/2$ cup	110	2%
yams and apples (Stouffer's)	5 oz	160	2%
Rice, white & spinach/cheese sauce,			
Italian blend (Green Giant Rice Orig)	$1/2$ cup	170	6%
Rice 'n broccoli in flavored cheese sauce			
Green Giant Rice Originals	$1/2$ cup	120	4%
Spinach			
Green Giant Harvest Fresh	$1/2$ cup	30	10%
Green Giant polybag	$1/2$ cup	25	10%
& water chestnuts (Birds Eye)	3.3 oz	25	8%
chopped (Birds Eye)	3.3 oz	20	10%
creamed (Birds Eye)	3 oz	60	8%
creamed (Green Giant)	$1/2$ cup	70	8%

Frozen vegetables: spinach *(continued)*

FOOD / BRAND NAME	SERVING	CALORIES	CALCIUM % U.S. RDA
souffle (Stouffer's)	4 oz	140	8%
whole leaf (Birds Eye)	3.3 oz	20	10%
Sweet corn (Birds Eye)	3.3 oz	80	*
Turnip greens, chopped (PictSweet)	3.2 oz	20	10%
Yams and apples (Stouffer's)	5 oz	160	2%

Grocery Department

Coffee creamers
Coffee-mate (Carnation)	1 tsp	10	*
Cremora (Borden)	1 tsp	12	*

Diet aids (prepared as directed on package)
Alba Fit 'n Frosty	1 envelope	70	30%
Alba '77 High Calcium Shake	1 envelope	70	30%
Carnation Slender			
bars, all flavors	2 bars	270	25%
liquid, all flavors	10 fl oz	220	25%
powdered mix, all flavors	1 envelope	200	25%

Instant drink mixes (prepared as directed on package)
Carnation Instant Breakfast			
chocolate	1 envelope	190	40%
chocolate malt	1 envelope	190	35%
strawberry	1 envelope	190	45%
vanilla	1 envelope	190	45%
Pillsbury: choc, choc malt, strawberry	1 pouch	290	25%
Pillsbury, vanilla	1 pouch	300	25%

Hot cocoa (prepared as directed on package)
Alba, all flavors	1 envelope	60	30%

* Less than 2% of the U.S. RDA

Hot cocoa *(continued)*

FOOD / BRAND NAME	SERVING	CALORIES	CALCIUM % U.S. RDA
Carnation			
milk chocolate	1 envelope	110	8%
mini marshmallow, rich chocolate	1 envelope	110	6%
rich chocolate, 70-calorie	1 envelope	70	10%
sugar free	1 envelope	50	10%
Ovaltine, hot 'n rich	1 envelope	120	10%
Swiss Miss			
double rich, mini marshmallow,			
milk chocolate	1 envelope	110	4%
sugar free	1 envelope	50	12%

Malted milk (prepared as directed on package)

Malted milk (Carnation)	3 tsp	90	6%
Malted milk, chocolate (Carnation)	3 tsp	79	*
Malted milk maker (Swiss Miss)	1 envelope	220	30%

Beans, canned

Baked beans			
B&M Brick Oven	8 oz	330	10%
Van Camp's	8 oz	260	10%
Barbecue beans (Campbell's)	$7^7/8$ oz	250	8%
Beanee Weenee (Van Camp's)	8 oz	330	8%
Brown sugar beans (Van Camp's)	8 oz	280	10%
Burrito filling mix (Del Monte)	1/2 cup	110	4%
Butter beans (Van Camp's)	8 oz	160	4%
Chilee Weenee (Van Camp's)	8 oz	310	6%
Chili beans (Hunt-Wesson)	4 oz	100	4%
Chili hot beans (Brooks)	1/2 cup	100	4%
Chili w/beans (Van Camp's)	8 oz	350	6%
Dark red & light kidney beans			
Van Camp's	8 oz	180	4%
Dark red kidney beans (Brooks)	1/2 cup	90	4%
Home style beans (Campbell's)	8 oz	270	10%

* Less than 2% of the U.S. RDA

Beans, canned *(continued)*

FOOD / BRAND NAME	SERVING	CALORIES	CALCIUM % U.S. RDA
Kidney beans			
dark red (Brooks)	¹/₂ cup	90	4%
dark red & light (Van Camp's)	8 oz	180	4%
New Orleans style (Van Camp's)	8 oz	180	4%
red (Hunt's)	4 oz	120	4%
Mexican style chili beans (Van Camp's)	8 oz	210	6%
New Orleans style kidney beans			
Van Camp's	8 oz	180	4%
Old fashioned beans in brown sugar			
& molasses sauce (Campbell's)	8 oz	270	10%
Pinto beans (Hanover)	1 cup	210	8%
Pork and beans			
Campbell's, in tomato sauce	8 oz	240	8%
Heinz	8 oz	250	15%
Hunt's	4 oz	140	4%
Libby's	1 cup	270	10%
Van Camp's	8 oz	220	8%
Red beans (Van Camp's)	8 oz	190	8%
Red kidney beans (Hunt's)	4 oz	120	4%
Refried beans (Del Monte)	¹/₂ cup	130	4%
Spicy refried beans (Del Monte)	¹/₂ cup	130	4%
Vegetarian, vegetarian style			
Heinz	8 oz	230	10%
Libby's	¹/₂ cup	260	10%
Van Camp's	8 oz	210	8%
Western style beans (Van Camp's)	8 oz	210	6%
Breads/English Muffins			
Bread (most types and brands)	1		2-4%
English muffins			
Bay's	1	140	8%
Merico	1	130	15%
Sun Maid Raisin	1	150	4%
Thomas			
plain	1	130	8%
honey wheat	1	130	2%
raisin	1	150	*

Cereals

FOOD / BRAND NAME	SERVING	CALORIES	CALCIUM % U.S. RDA

Cereals

A major calcium-boosting benefit of breakfast cereal is the milk that you pour over it. Just a half-cup of milk adds 15% of the U.S. RDA for calcium, whether the milk is skim, lowfat, or whole. The following cereals contain over 2% of the U.S. RDA for calcium.

COLD CEREALS

FOOD / BRAND NAME	SERVING	CALORIES	CALCIUM % U.S. RDA
All Bran fruit & almonds (Kellogg's)	1 oz	100	4%
Body Buddies, brown sugar & honey/ fruit flavor (General Mills)	1 oz	110	10%
Bran Muffin Crisp (General Mills)	1.4 oz	130	6%
Cheerios (General Mills)	1 oz	110	4%
Cinnamon Life (Quaker)	1 oz	120	6%
Cinnamon Toast Crunch (General Mills)	1 oz	120	4%
Crispy Wheats 'n Raisins (General Mills)	1 oz	110	4%
Fiber One (General Mills)	1 oz	60	6%
Honey Buc Wheat Crisp (General Mills)	1 oz	110	6%
Kix (General Mills)	1 oz	110	4%
Life (Quaker)	1 oz	120	6%
100% natural apple & cinnamon (Quaker)	1 oz	130	4%
Raisin Life (Quaker)	1 oz	150	6%
Raisin Nut Bran (General Mills)	1 oz	110	4%
Total corn flakes (General Mills)	1 oz	110	20%
Total whole wheat (General Mills)	1 oz	100	20%
Wheaties (General Mills)	1 oz	110	4%

HOT CEREALS

FOOD / BRAND NAME	SERVING	CALORIES	CALCIUM % U.S. RDA
Oatmeal, instant (Quaker)			
regular flavor	1 packet	100	10%
apples/cinnamon	1 packet	130	10%
bran/raisins	1 packet	150	10%
honey/graham	1 packet	140	10%
maple/brown sugar	1 packet	160	10%
peaches/cream	1 packet	140	10%
raisins/spice	1 packet	160	10%
strawberries/cream	1 packet	140	10%

* Less than 2% U.S. RDA

Cereals, hot *(continued)*

FOOD / BRAND NAME	SERVING	CALORIES	CALCIUM % U.S. RDA
Oatmeal, instant (Total)			
cinnamon raisin almond	1 packet	160	20%
regular flavor	1 packet	100	20%
Oatmeal, 30-sec. maple flavor (May-Po)	1 oz	123	8%
Wheat (Cream of Wheat)			
instant, quick, regular, & mix 'n eat	1 oz	100	4%

Entrees, packaged *(prepared as directed)*

FOOD / BRAND NAME	SERVING	CALORIES	CALCIUM % U.S. RDA
Alfredo noodles & sauce (Lipton Deluxe)	$1/2$ cup	220	10%
Beef romanoff (Hamburger Helper)	$1/5$ pkg	350	6%
Cheeseburger macaroni			
Hamburger Helper	$1/5$ pkg	360	6%
Cheese noodles & sauce (Lipton Deluxe)	$1/2$ cup	200	4%
Egg noodle & cheese dinner (Kraft)	$3/4$ cup	340	10%
Egg noodle w/chicken dinner (Kraft)	$3/4$ cup	240	4%
Elbow macaroni & cheese			
Franco-American	$7 3/8$ oz	170	8%
Fettucine alfredo noodle mix			
Betty Crocker	$1/4$ pkg	230	15%
Hamburger Mate burger 'n cheese			
dinner (Creamette)	$1/5$ pkg	170	10%
Lasagna dinner (Chef Boyardee)	5.9 oz	290	10%
Macaroni & cheese			
Borden	2 oz	220	10%
Creamettes	$3/4$ cup	300	10%
Franco-American	$7 3/8$ oz	170	8%
Franco-American, elbow mac.	$7 3/8$ oz	170	8%
Kraft	$3/4$ cup	290	8%
Kraft Deluxe	$3/4$ cup	260	10%
Parmesano noodles/sauce (Lipton Deluxe)	$1/2$ cup	210	6%
Romanoff noodle mix (Betty Crocker)	$1/4$ pkg	220	6%
Shells and cheese (Kraft Velveeta)	$3/4$ cup	260	20%
Welsh rarebit cheese sauce (Snow's)	$1/2$ cup	170	25%

Fruit, dried *(see Produce)*

Legumes, dry (cooked)

FOOD / BRAND NAME	SERVING	CALORIES	CALCIUM % U.S. RDA
Legumes, dry (cooked)			
Great Northern beans	1 cup	210	9%
Lentils	1 cup	215	5%
Pea beans (navy)	1 cup	225	10%
Pinto beans	1 cup	265	8%
Red kidney beans	1 cup	230	7%
Milk, dry and canned			
Instant low fat dry milk (Carnation)	8 fl oz*	90	29%
Instant nonfat dry milk			
Alba	8 fl oz*	80	30%
Carnation	8 fl oz*	80	30%
Flash	8 fl oz*	80	30%
Sanalac	$1/4$ env*	80	30%
Evaporated milk			
Carnation	4 fl oz	170	30%
Carnation, low fat	4 fl oz	110	30%
Carnation, skimmed	4 fl oz	100	35%
Gold Cross	$1/2$ cup	170	30%
Pet	$1/2$ cup	170	30%
Sweetened condensed milk			
Eagle	$1/3$ cup	320	30%
Magnolia	$1/3$ cup	320	30%
Pancake and Waffle Mixes *(4" pancakes prepared as directed on package)*			
Blueberry (Hungry Jack)	3	320	10%
Buckwheat (Aunt Jemima)	3	200	15%
Buttermilk			
Aunt Jemima	3	300	30%
Betty Crocker	3	280	15%
Hungry Jack	3	240	6%
Buttermilk complete			
Aunt Jemima	3	260	40%
Betty Crocker	3	210	10%
Hungry Jack	3	180	15%
Mrs. Butterworth's	3	195	15%

* Reconstituted with water

Pancake and waffle mixes (*continued*)

FOOD / BRAND NAME	SERVING	CALORIES	CALCIUM % U.S. RDA
Complete			
Aunt Jemima	3	280	10%
Extra Lights Hungry Jack	3	190	10%
Extra Lights (Hungry Jack)	3	210	15%
Golden Blend (Hungry Jack)	3	200	15%
Golden Blend complete (Hungry Jack)	3	240	15%
Old Fashioned (Mrs. Butterworth's)	3	140	30%
Original (Aunt Jemima)	3	220	15%
Panshakes (Hungry Jack)	3	250	15%
Whole wheat (Aunt Jemima)	3	250	20%

Pudding, canned

FOOD / BRAND NAME	SERVING	CALORIES	CALCIUM % U.S. RDA
Banana			
Del Monte pudding cup	5 oz	180	10%
Hunt's snack pack	5 oz	210	4%
Butterscotch			
Del Monte pudding cup	5 oz	180	10%
Hunt's snack pack	5 oz	210	4%
Chocolate			
Del Monte pudding cup	5 oz	190	10%
Hunt's snack pack	5 oz	210	4%
Chocolate fudge			
Del Monte pudding cup	5 oz	190	10%
Hunt's snack pack	5 oz	200	2%
Chocolate marshmallow			
Hunt's snack pack	5 oz	200	*
German chocolate (Hunt's snack pack)	5 oz	220	*
Lemon (Hunt's snack pack)	5 oz	180	*
Rice (Hunt's snack pack)	5 oz	220	6%
Tapioca			
Del Monte pudding cup	5 oz	180	10%
Hunt's snack pack	5 oz	140	6%
Vanilla			
Del Monte pudding cup	5 oz	180	10%
Hunt's snack pack	5 oz	210	4%

* Less than 2% U.S. RDA

Snacks, packaged

FOOD / BRAND NAME	SERVING	CALORIES	CALCIUM % U.S. RDA
Snacks, packaged			
Almonds, dry, roasted (Planters)	1 oz	170	8%
Cheez 'n crackers (Handi-Snacks)	1 pkg	120	10%
Cheddar sticks (Flavor Tree)	1 oz	160	6%
Cheez waffies (Wise)	1 oz	140	6%
Combos, pretzels/pizza/nacho flavors	1.8 oz	240	10%
Combos, pretzels (Cheddar)	1.8 oz	240	8%
Sesame Chips/Sticks (Flavor Tree)	1 oz	150	6%
Smoked Almonds (Planters)	1 oz	170	6%
Vegetables, canned			
Collard greens (Allens)	1/2 cup	25	10%
Mustard greens (Allens)	1/2 cup	20	10%
Spinach, cut leaf (Freshlike)	1/2 cup	25	8%
Spinach, whole leaf (Del Monte)	1/2 cup	25	10%
Turnip greens, chopped (Allens)	1/2 cup	25	10%
Fish, canned			
Oysters (Bumble Bee)	1/2 cup	100	2%
Salmon			
blueback (Bumble Bee)	3.5 oz	180	15%
pink (Bumble Bee)	3.5 oz	160	20%
red sockeye (Bumble Bee)	3.5 oz	180	15%
Sardines			
Del Monte, in tomato sauce	7 1/2 oz	380	100%
Spirit of Norway, w/skin & bones	3 3/4 oz	260	30%
Underwood/soya oil	3 oz	230	25%

Produce Department

Fruit, fresh

Apple	1	81	*
Apricots	3	51	*
Banana	1	105	*

* Less than 2% U.S. RDA

Fresh fruit *(continued)*

FOOD / BRAND NAME	SERVING	CALORIES	CALCIUM % U.S. RDA
Blackberries	1/2 cup	37	2%
Blueberries	1/2 cup	41	*
Cantaloupe, 5" diam.	1/2	94	3%
Cherries	10	49	*
Fig	1 large	47	2%
Grapes, seedless	10	36	*
Honeydew melon	1/10 melon	46	*
Orange	1	62	5%
Orange juice, fresh	1 cup	111	3%
Papaya	1	117	7%
Peach	1	37	*
Pear, Bartlett	1	98	2%
Pineapple, diced	1 cup	77	*
Plum	1	36	*
Rhubarb, diced	1/2 cup	13	5%
Strawberries	1 cup	45	2%
Tangerine	1	37	*
Watermelon, wedge	1" x 10"	152	4%

Fruit, dried

Apricots, large	7 halves	77	*
Dates	10	230	3%
Figs	10	475	27%
Peaches	1/4 cup	95	*
Prunes	5 large	115	2%
Raisins, seedless (packed)	1/4 cup	109	*

* Less than 2% U.S. RDA

Nuts and seeds

FOOD / BRAND NAME	SERVING	CALORIES	CALCIUM % U.S. RDA
Nuts and seeds			
Almonds, whole	1 oz	165	7%
Brazil nuts, shelled	1 oz	185	5%
Cashews, roasted in oil	1 oz	165	*
Filberts (hazelnuts)	1 oz	180	5%
Peanuts, roasted in oil	1 oz	160	3%
Sesame seeds, dry, hulled	1 Tbsp	45	*
Sunflower seeds, dry, hulled	1 oz	160	3%
Walnuts, black	1 oz	170	*
Walnuts, English	1 oz	180	3%

Tofu

The U.S. Dept. of Agriculture Home and Garden Bulletin #72 (1981) lists the following nutritional data on tofu:

Tofu (piece 2 $\frac{1}{2}$" x 2 $\frac{3}{4}$" x 1")	85	10%

The calories and calcium in tofu are actually extremely variable. The calories may range between 60-130 for a 4-ounce serving. Tofu that is coagulated with calcium sulfate or calcium chloride usually ranges between 15%-30% of the U.S. RDA for calcium. When tofu is coagulated with nigari only, the calcium content is likely to be less than 5%.

Vegetables, fresh Cooked (boiled & drained) unless indicated as raw

Asparagus	4 spears	15	*
Beans, lima	$\frac{1}{2}$ cup	104	3%
Beans, snap	$\frac{1}{2}$ cup	22	3%
Beet greens	$\frac{1}{2}$ cup	20	8%
Beets, sliced	$\frac{1}{2}$ cup	26	*
Bok choy, shredded	$\frac{1}{2}$ cup	10	8%
Broccoli, chopped	$\frac{1}{2}$ cup	23	9%
Brussels sprouts	$\frac{1}{2}$ cup	30	3%

* Less than 2% U.S. RDA

Fresh vegetables *(continued)*

FOOD / BRAND NAME	SERVING	CALORIES	CALCIUM % U.S. RDA
Carrots, raw, sliced	1/2 cup	35	2%
Cauliflower	3 flowerets	13	*
Celery, raw, diced	1/2 cup	9	2%
Chard, swiss (*see* Swiss chard)			
Chinese cabbage (*see* Bok choy)			
Collards, chopped	1/2 cup	13	7%
Corn	1 ear	83	*
Cucumber, raw, sliced	1/2 cup	7	*
Dandelion greens, chopped	1/2 cup	17	7%
raw, chopped	1/2 cup	13	5%
Eggplant, 1" cubes	1/2 cup	13	*
Green onions, raw, chopped	1/2 cup	13	3%
Kale, chopped	1/2 cup	20	5%
Kale, Scotch, chopped	1/2 cup	18	8%
Kohlrabi, sliced	1/2 cup	24	2%
Lettuce, romaine, raw, shredded	1/2 cup	4	*
Mushrooms, raw, cut in pieces	1/2 cup	9	*
Mustard greens, chopped	1/2 cup	11	5%
Okra, sliced	1/2 cup	25	5%
Spinach, raw, chopped	1/2 cup	6	3%
Spinach	1/2 cup	21	12%
Swiss chard	1/2 cup	18	5%
Turnip greens, chopped	1/2 cup	15	10%

* Less than 2% of the U.S. RDA

12

CALCIUM AND CALORIE COUNTER
FOR
FAST FOOD RESTAURANTS

MANY FAST FOOD restaurants have responded to the needs of health-conscious consumers by adding salads or salad bars, as well as low fat and/or skim milk. When making menu choices, cheese is the key to calcium: in cheeseburgers, fish/cheese sandwiches, cheese-stuffed potatoes, omelets with cheese, and Mexican specialties.

The calcium and calories of foods at nine popular fast food restaurants are given here. The nutritional data has been provided by each restaurant chain.

Arby's
Burger King
Dairy Queen
Jack in the Box
McDonald's
Rax
Roy Rogers
Taco Bell
Wendy's

Arby's

Entrees

	CAL-ORIES	CALCIUM U.S. RDA
Bac'n cheddar deluxe	526	15%
Beef 'n cheddar	455	6%
Chicken breast sandwich	509	8%
Hot ham 'n cheese	292	20%
Roast beef		
Giant	531	10%
Junior	218	4%
King	467	10%
Phylly beef 'n swiss	460	45%
Regular	353	8%
Super	501	10%
Turkey deluxe	375	8%

Side dishes

	CAL-ORIES	CALCIUM U.S. RDA
French fries	215	*
Potato cakes	201	*

Beverages, desserts

	CAL-ORIES	CALCIUM U.S. RDA
Shake, chocolate	451	25%
Shake, jamocha	368	25%
Shake, vanilla	330	30%
Turnover, apple	303	*
Turnover, cherry	280	2%

* Less than 2% U.S. RDA

Burger King

Breakfast

	CAL-ORIES	CALCIUM U.S. RDA
Breakfast Croissan'wich		
Bacon, egg, cheese	355	14%
Ham, egg, cheese	335	14%
Sausage, egg, cheese	538	15%
French toast sticks	499	8%
Great Danish	500	9%
Scrambled egg platter	468	10%
w/bacon	536	10%
w/sausage	702	11%

Beverages, desserts

Apple pie	305	*
Chocolate shake	320	26%
w/syrup added	374	25%
Milk, 2% lowfat	121	30%
Milk, whole	157	29%
Vanilla shake	321	29%

Entrees

	CAL-ORIES	CALCIUM U.S. RDA
Bacon double cheeseburger	510	17%
Cheeseburger	317	10%
Chicken sandwich	688	8%
Chicken tenders (6 pc.)	204	2%
Hamburger	275	4%
Ham & cheese sandwich	471	19%
Whaler sandwich	488	5%
Whopper sandwich	628	8%
Whopper w/cheese	711	21%
Whopper, jr. sandwich	322	4%
Whopper, jr. w/cheese	364	11%

Side dishes

French fries	227	*
Onion rings	274	12%

* Less than 2% U.S. RDA

Dairy Queen

Entrees	CAL-ORIES	CALCIUM U.S. RDA
Chicken breast fillet	608	15%
w/cheese	661	25%
DQ sandwich	140	6%
Fish fillet	430	15%
w/cheese	483	25%
Hamburger, single	360	10%
w/cheese	410	20%
Hamburger, double	530	10%
w/cheese	650	35%
Hamburger, triple	710	10%
w/cheese	820	35%
Hot dog, regular	280	8%
w/cheese	330	15%
w/chili	320	8%
Hot dog, super	520	15%
w/cheese	580	25%
w/chili	570	15%

Side dishes

	CAL-ORIES	CALCIUM U.S. RDA
French fries		
regular	200	*
large	320	2%
Onion rings	280	10%

* Less than 2% U.S. RDA

Beverages, desserts	CAL-ORIES	CALCIUM U.S. RDA
Banana split	540	25%
Buster bar	460	10%
"Chipper" sandwich	318	10%
Cone		
small	140	10%
regular	240	15%
large	340	25%
Dilly bar	210	10%
Dipped cone, chocolate		
small	190	10%
regular	340	15%
large	520	25%
Double delight	490	20%
Float	410	20%
Heath blizzard (16 oz)	800	50%
Hot fudge brownie delight	600	20%
Malt, chocolate		
small	520	35%
regular	760	45%
large (21 oz)	889	55%
Mr. Misty float	390	20%
Mr. Misty freeze	500	30%
Parfait	430	25%
Peanut butter parfait	740	25%
Shake, chocolate		
small	490	35%
regular	710	45%
large (21 oz)	831	55%
Strawberry shortcake	540	25%
Sundae, chocolate		
small	190	10%
regular	310	20%
large	440	25%

Jack in the Box

Breakfast

	CAL-ORIES	CALCIUM U.S. RDA
Breakfast Jack	307	17%
Canadian crescent	452	13%
Pancake platter	612	10%
Sausage crescent	584	17%
Scrambled egg platter	662	20%
Supreme crescent	547	15%

Entrees

	CAL-ORIES	CALCIUM U.S. RDA
Bacon cheeseburger	705	28%
Cheeseburger	325	6%
Chicken strip dinner (without sauce)	674	8%
Chicken supreme sandwich	575	10%
Fajita pita (no sauce)	277	30%
Hamburger	288	4%
Ham 'n swiss burger	754	28%
Jumbo Jack	584	14%
w/cheese	677	27%
Moby Jack	444	16%
Monterey burger	808	27%
Mushroom burger	470	25%
Nachos		
cheese	571	37%
supreme	639	20%
Pizza pocket	497	10%
Shrimp dinner (without sauce)	677	30%

Entrees (cont.)

	CAL-ORIES	CALCIUM U.S. RDA
Sirloin steak dinner (without sauce)	702	20%
Swiss & bacon burger	678	22%
Taco		
regular	191	10%
super	288	15%

Side dishes, salads

	CAL-ORIES	CALCIUM U.S. RDA
Chef salad	295	15%
Pasta & seafood salad	394	21%
Side salad	51	6%
Taco salad	377	28%
French fries		
regular	221	*
large	353	*
Onion rings	382	3%

Beverages, desserts

	CAL-ORIES	CALCIUM U.S. RDA
Apple turnover	410	*
Cheesecake	309	11%
Chocolate shake	330	35%
Milk, lowfat	122	30%
Orange juice	80	2%
Shake		
strawberry	320	35%
vanilla	320	35%

* Less than 2% U.S. RDA

McDonald's

Breakfast

	CAL-ORIES	CALCIUM U.S. RDA
Biscuit	330	8%
w/bacon, egg & cheese	483	*
w/sausage	467	8%
w/sausage & egg	585	10%
Danish		
apple	389	*
cheese	395	4%
cinnamon raisin	445	4%
raspberry	414	*
Egg McMuffin	340	25%
English muffin		
w/butter	186	10%
Hash brown potatoes	144	*
Hotcakes w/butter & syrup	500	10%
Sausage	210	*
Sausage McMuffin	427	15%
w/egg	517	20%
Scrambled eggs	180	6%

Entrees

Big Mac	570	20%
Cheeseburger	318	15%
Chicken McNuggets	323	*
Filet-O-Fish	435	15%
Hamburger	263	8%
Mc D.L.T.	680	25%
Quarter Pounder	427	10%
w/cheese	525	25%

Side dishes, salads

	CAL-ORIES	CALCIUM U.S. RDA
French fries	220	*
Chef salad	226	20%
Chicken salad oriental	146	4%
Garden salad	91	10%
Shrimp salad	99	6%
Side salad	48	4%

Beverages, desserts

Apple pie	253	*
Cones, soft serve	189	20%
Milk		
skim	90	30%
2%	121	30%
Milk shake		
chocolate	383	30%
strawberry	362	30%
vanilla	352	30%
Sundae		
hot caramel	361	20%
hot fudge	357	20%
strawberry	320	15%

* Less than 2% U.S. RDA

Rax

Sandwiches

	CAL-ORIES	CALCIUM U.S. RDA
Barbecue beef	350	4%
Beef, bacon, cheddar	670	2%
Chicken	580	2%
Ham 'n cheese	350	15%
Roast beef	370	2%
Philly beef 'n cheese	510	15%
Turkey bacon club	570	2%

Potatoes

	CAL-ORIES	CALCIUM U.S. RDA
Bacon/cheese skins	95	4%
Bacon/cheese	590	20%
Beef barbecue	720	4%
Beef stroganoff	540	8%
Broccoli/cheese	560	25%
French fries	340	2%
Mexican	610	18%
Pizza	470	15%

Beverages, desserts

	CAL-ORIES	CALCIUM U.S. RDA
Chocolate chip cookie (1)	130	14%
Shake		
chocolate	470	40%
strawberry	470	40%
vanilla	450	40%

Roy Rogers

Breakfast

	CAL-ORIES	CALCIUM U.S. RDA
Crescent sandwich	401	16%
w/bacon	431	16%
w/ham	557	16%
w/sausage	449	16%
Egg & biscuit platter	394	12%
w/bacon	435	12%
w/ham	442	12%
w/sausage	550	12%
Pancake platter (syrup and butter)	452	9%
w/bacon	493	9%
w/ham	506	9%
w/sausage	608	9%

Entrees

Bacon cheeseburger	581	34%
Cheeseburger	563	34%
Chicken breast	412	2%
and wing	604	2%
Chicken leg	117	*
Chicken thigh	296	*
and leg	436	3%
Roast beef sandwich	317	8%
with cheese	424	34%
Roast beef sand., large	360	9%
with cheese	467	34%
RR Bar Burger	611	34%

Hot topped potatoes

	CAL-ORIES	CALCIUM U.S. RDA
Plain	211	2%
w/bacon & cheese	397	15%
w/broccoli & cheese	376	21%
w/oleo	274	2%
w/sour cream/chives	408	9%
w/taco beef & cheese	463	15%

Side dishes, salads

Cole slaw	110	3%
French fries		
regular	268	*
large	357	2%
Macaroni	186	*
Potato salad	107	*

Beverages, desserts

Danish		
apple	249	10%
cherry	271	4%
cheese	254	4%
Brownie	264	2%
Hot chocolate	123	8%
Milk	150	30%
Shake		
chocolate	358	29%
strawberry	315	28%
Sundae		
caramel	293	20%
hot fudge	337	26%
strawberry	216	21%

* Less than 2% U.S. RDA

Taco Bell

Burritos

	CALORIES	CALCIUM U.S. RDA
Bean	360	12%
green	354	11%
Beef	402	10%
green	396	9%
Combo	381	11%
green	375	10%
Double beef supreme	464	14%
green	459	13%
Supreme	422	14%
green	416	13%
Supreme platter	774	31%
green	762	29%

Nachos, beans & pizza

Nachos	356	18%
bellgrande	719	32%
Pintos & cheese	194	14%
green	188	13%
Pizzazz pizza	714	45%

Tacos

	CALORIES	CALCIUM U.S. RDA
Taco	184	8%
Bellgrande	350	16%
platter	1001	47%
platter, green	990	45%
Light	411	15%
platter	1062	46%
platter, green	1050	44%
Soft	228	11%

Salads

Seafood salad	920	32%
without shell	223	25%
without dressing	648	29%
Taco salad	949	39%
without beans	820	35%
without shell	523	35%
w/ ranch dressing	1204	39%

Wendy's

Breakfast

	CAL-ORIES	CALCIUM U.S. RDA
Bacon (strip)	30	*
Breakfast potatoes	360	2%
Breakfast sandwich	370	15%
Buttermilk biscuit	320	10%
Danish		
apple	360	6%
cheese	430	8%
cinnamon raisin	410	6%
Egg, fried	90	2%
Eggs, scrambled	190	6%
French toast	400	8%
Omelets		
Ham & cheese	290	10%
Ham, cheese and mushroom	250	10%
Ham, cheese, onion & green pepper	280	15%
Mushroom, green pepper and onion	210	6%

Entrees

Bacon cheeseburger	455	19%
Big Classic	470	4%
Big Classic double	680	4%
Chicken club sandwich	479	*
Chicken filet sandwich	340	*
Chili	240	6%
Crispy chicken nuggets	310	2%
Fish sandwich	430	*
Kids meal hamburger	270	4%
Single hamburger	350	4%
Taco salad	430	30%

Side dishes

	CAL-ORIES	CALCIUM U.S. RDA
French fries	310	*
Salad bar *(only items with over 2% U.S. RDA for calcium are listed)*		
American cheese (imitation), 1 oz	90	20%
Cheddar cheese (imitation), 1 oz	80	20%
Cottage cheese, 1/2 cup	110	6%
Mozzarella cheese (imitation), 1 oz	90	20%
Swiss cheese (imitation), 1 oz	90	20%
Stuffed baked potatoes		
cheese	590	35%
& bacon	570	20%
& broccoli	500	25%
& chili	510	25%
plain	250	4%
sour cream & chives	460	4%

Beverages, desserts

Frosty dairy dessert	400	30%
Hot chocolate	110	6%
Milk		
chocolate	190	25%
2%	110	30%
whole	140	25%

* Less than 2% U.S. RDA